THE
EVERYTHING
EASY CLEANSE
BOOK

Dear Reader,

One day during a short religious fast, a type of total cleanse of my every-day life, I was thinking about the meaning of body strength versus fragil-ity. As this cleanse period was ending, I walked into my mother's new garden to smell the clean green of the leaves and vines. The colors of the vegetables themselves had an aroma of spicy red, honeying yellows, earthy purples, and cool dewy greens. I reached into the thorny black-berry bush and tasted a finger-staining, juicy berry, so powerful in its natural coloring abilities despite its the tender form. A handful of tiny yel-low tomatoes had instant taste and smell sensations with no artificial bar-rier to the skin. This cleansing period brought me to focus on not filling up my body to satisfy whims or indulgences, but a knowingness of some truths about what will help keep my body protected and healthy.

You too can have your own personal "a-ha" experience about ridding yourself of bad stuff and keeping your body healthfully protected. Make a small space and time in your life that separates and leaves behind your typical lifestyle to cleanse yourself of yesterday's misguided choices, excesses, or just to discover some more truths. This is an opportunity to learn more about what you can do to help your body keep nasty invaders, toxins, and other bad stuff at bay, and keep yourself as strong and healthy as you deserve to be. I invite you to give yourself that opportunity.

Cynthia Lechan Goodman

Welcome to the EVERYTHING® Series!

These handy, accessible books give you all you need to tackle a difficult project, gain a new hobby, comprehend a fascinating topic, prepare for an exam, or even brush up on something you learned back in school but have since forgotten.

You can choose to read an *Everything®* book from cover to cover or just pick out the information you want from our four useful boxes: e-questions, e-facts, e-alerts, and e-ssentials.

We give you everything you need to know on the subject, but throw in a lot of fun stuff along the way, too.

We now have more than 400 *Everything®* books in print, spanning such wide-ranging categories as weddings, pregnancy, cooking, music instruction, foreign language, crafts, pets, New Age, and so much more. When you're done reading them all, you can finally say you know *Everything®*!

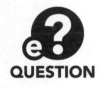

QUESTION

Answers to
common questions

FACT

Important snippets
of information

ALERT

Urgent
warnings

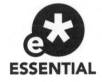

ESSENTIAL

Quick
handy tips

PUBLISHER Karen Cooper

DIRECTOR OF ACQUISITIONS AND INNOVATION Paula Munier

MANAGING EDITOR, EVERYTHING® SERIES Lisa Laing

COPY CHIEF Casey Ebert

ASSISTANT PRODUCTION EDITOR Jacob Erickson

ACQUISITIONS EDITOR Kate Powers

SENIOR DEVELOPMENT EDITOR Brett Palana-Shanahan

EDITORIAL ASSISTANT Ross Weisman

EVERYTHING® SERIES COVER DESIGNER Erin Alexander

LAYOUT DESIGNERS Colleen Cunningham, Elisabeth Lariviere, Ashley Vierra, Denise Wallace

Visit the entire Everything® series at *www.everything.com*

THE EVERYTHING® EASY CLEANSE BOOK

Recipes, tips, and tricks for
a safe and healthy detox!

Cynthia Lechan Goodman
Nutrition Expert on Blend.com

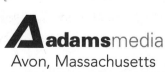

Avon, Massachusetts

To my darling daughter, Lailee Natane.
May opportunities for your many talents to
shine keep coming your way, and may you
enjoy it all—always in the peak of health and
surrounded by loving family and friends.

An Everything® Series Book.
Everything® and everything.com® are registered trademarks of F+W Media, Inc.

Published by Adams Media, a division of F+W Media, Inc.
57 Littlefield Street, Avon, MA 02322 U.S.A.
www.adamsmedia.com

ISBN 10: 1-4405-2502-1
ISBN 13: 978-1-4405-2502-5
eISBN 10: 1-4405-2547-1
eISBN 13: 978-1-4405-2547-6

Printed in the United States of America.

10 9 8 7 6 5 4 3 2 1

Library of Congress Cataloging-in-Publication Data
is available from the publisher.

The information in this book should not be used for diagnosing or treating any health problem. Not all diet and exercise plans suit everyone. You should always consult a trained medical professional before starting a diet, taking any form of medication, or embarking on any fitness or weight-training program. The author and publisher disclaim any liability arising directly or indirectly from the use of this book.

This publication is designed to provide accurate and authoritative information with regard to the subject matter covered. It is sold with the understanding that the publisher is not engaged in rendering legal, accounting, or other professional advice. If legal advice or other expert assistance is required, the services of a competent professional person should be sought.

—From a *Declaration of Principles* jointly adopted by a Committee of the American Bar Association and a Committee of Publishers and Associations

Many of the designations used by manufacturers and sellers to distinguish their products are claimed as trademarks. Where those designations appear in this book and Adams Media was aware of a trademark claim, the designations have been printed with initial capital letters.

This book is available at quantity discounts for bulk purchases.
For information, please call 1-800-289-0963.

Contents

Acknowledgments

With loving admiration and thankfulness to my father, Dr. Harry Lechan, for inspiring me with his passion for knowledge, health, and family. From his days of making house calls for sick babies at night with a chicken as payment, until today at ninety-five, he always advocates, "when you have your health, you have everything."

With loving appreciation and thankfulness to my mother, Sylvia, for inspiring me with her tireless devotion to nurturing her family for sixty years with balanced nutrition, healing soups, gardens of beautiful flowers and produce, a positive outlook, and an interest in the good things people do.

With infinite loving thankfulness to my supportive husband, Steve, for his devotion to me.

With special love and thankfulness to my brothers Ronnie, Alan, and Laurence for always cheering me on as a hero.

With grateful appreciation to Gayle Stolove, owner of *www .whollymacrobiotics.com*, for sharing her professional knowledge in holistic and Oriental health care and food and beverage recipes, some of which are included in this book.

A heartfelt thank-you to my editor Kate Powers for her caring concern, warm encouragement, and for my good fortune to have the benefits of her talents and knowledge.

Top 10 Helpers for
Healthy Bodily Cleansing

1. Green tea, cinnamon, or natural fruit-flavored teas are all a boon for any cleanse and healthy diet.

2. Protein-rich, calcium-rich, nutrient-rich cottage cheese is great for many cleansing daily plans.

3. Antioxidant fruits like plums—fresh or dried as a prune.

4. Water—and plenty of it—is essential to cleansing the body and healthy living.

5. Eat your eggs! In liquid in a shake or smoothie, hard-boiled, or scrambled, you are getting excellent recommended daily nutrients for cleansing and health.

6. Green, black, or red, beans are nutrient-rich foods for any cleansing diet and for daily health.

7. Complex carbs, protein, and fiber are most important for cleansing and daily health.

8. Pumpkin with its brilliant vitamin A, beta-carotene, and other great nutrients, is wonderful for cleansing and daily health.

9. When you want to do the best for your bodily cleansing and health, you need to get enough sleep.

10. An apple a day keeps the doctor away, and cancer, and heart disease, and any number of other nasty conditions!

Introduction

NOT ALWAYS FEELING SO great? Blues, sniffles, congestion, aches, foggy brain, tired, pimply reflection in the mirror, bloated, constipated, weak with no energy, irritable? At times like these people are often in a quandary, wondering "what should I do for myself to get rid of this badness—to cleanse it out, and not only get rid of it, but also prevent it from coming back? Should I go for fizzy ginger ale, chicken soup, chocolate cake, or what?"

Not feeling so great seems to be happening to us too often. And you have very real worries hearing daily news reports that toxins in food, medications, and the environment are getting into your body and can be contributing to a lot of this ill health. You may have also been hearing about the idea of cleansing—something you can do to help your body deal with this bad stuff. But if you are a little cautious, and curious, and want to be in the know about cleansing and your health, you are right to be reading this book—so that you *won't* be in such a quandary wondering what and how and when to do something good for your health. That's what this book is all about. Chapters related to your own issues will help you to find out what kind of cleansing path you might decide to take. All of the cleansing paths described in this book have great body-gratifying foods with nutrients that will help your body deal with and prevent those invaders and toxins doing their nasty work that makes you feel lousy.

Using a cleansing path to healing is not just a random idea found on the Internet, but has been practiced throughout history. Hippocrates, a Greek physician in the fifth and fourth century B.C. who is considered to be the father of medicine, is claimed to have said, "The natural healing force within each one of us is the greatest force in getting well. Our food should be our medicine." Records about his methods describe that for some fevers and diseases he prescribed a fasting type of cleanse—using water or teas, or a small diet of thin or liquid foods.

While scientific research is limited on cleansing diets, there is an overwhelming amount of personal accounts and professional proponents of the health benefits of cleansing paths for diets. These benefits include better digestion and mental function, better energy, better skin, better management of weight issues, better moods, and better general health, vitality, and resistance to illnesses.

There is beauty in cleansing. Unfortunately, many people incorrectly think cleansing is only about the colon—and that may not bring about especially beautiful thoughts! But that is because a focus on the colon is only about an end, and what comes out—and when it comes to cleansing, your focus should be on the beginning and what goes in! As you will see in *The Everything® Easy Cleanse Book*, cleansing is a path to your health, and this book will tell you all about the best-known nutrients for you to begin the process. You will find out all the easy information about them, how and where to get them, and how to use them in a diet that is right for you to put them to work on your personal cleansing path to better health. Each chapter takes you through the steps describing the area of your issues, how they might come about, what particular nutrients the body uses in maintaining better health in these areas, what foods have these nutrients, and an easy procedure for developing your cleansing path for your issues.

Recipe suggestions are given and suggestions for before, during, and after a cleanse period. The information passed along to you about nutrients, foods, and the body systems are taken from many documented and published medical studies from universities and research facilities all over the world, and from published opinions of medical professionals and well-known nutritional experts.

Cleansing is about the beginnings of a journey to a new and healthier you. Since you are reading this book, you are already in the know about taking steps to make a change in your health for the better. *The Everything® Easy Cleanse Book* will take the mystery out of the realm of cleansing for you. You will be able to easily learn about types of cleanses, what you need to know to feel safe about the choices you make, what cleanses are directed to your issues, why certain nutrients and foods will help your issues, and how to make an easy path for yourself toward your own goals for your health.

CHAPTER 1

To Cleanse or Not to Cleanse

Since you were a kid you've been fighting off dragons, giants, dinosaurs, and witches who want to poison you with apples, burn you up with fire breath, eat you alive, or fling you onto the rocks. And now that you're an adult, there are still monsters out to attack you. They are in the form of toxins, illnesses, and diseases that grab you and hold you down. These monsters are no fairy tales; they are real, but the good news is you don't need to be a knight in shining armor to get rid of them. In fact, it's as simple as the way you make sure to clean your hands and face to keep yourself fresh, healthy, and germ-free. What you can do for the outside, you can also easily and safely do for the *inside*, and clear out the "bogeymen" that want to rob you of great health, energy, and clear thinking.

Why Are You Cleansing?

When you were a kid you probably thought you'd live forever, and there wasn't too much that got you to worry about your body—after all, your body was always there doing its job. Well, in fact, the body does go on doing the job it is supposed to do, but nowadays, you feel tired, exhausted, sick, pains here and there, and a host of other things in the body that you wish would disappear. The news reports all talk about the toxins that get into your body from the environment, the air, the water, and from highly processed foods that are loaded with chemicals and nonfood additives.

So why are you cleansing? Think about it. Do you want to lose some of that holiday weight? Have you had trouble with digestion? Feeling anxious all the time? Just want to clean it all out and start fresh? When you consider the reasons behind your cleanse, it can help you determine which program you should use on your journey. You need goals for your cleanse to be successful, so "just wanting to do one" is not a very good reason. Really take the time to consider what you want from your nutrient cleanse; sometimes making a goal list is helpful. That way you have it on paper so you can measure your outcomes after the cleanse is complete.

As always, when you finally determine your reasons for cleansing, consult your doctor before beginning to ensure that you have no physical or mental issues that can interfere with (or be interfered by) your cleanse.

What Does a Cleanse Do for the Body?

The human body has an amazing natural cleansing system for getting rid of toxins. The body's natural cleansing machinery is made up of several systems that work together: the liver, the kidneys, the colon, the lungs, and the skin. In some way all of these organs are involved in the processing of nutrients and the elimination of wastes and toxins. The better you treat them with good nutrients, the better they will be able to do their jobs of cleansing the body.

In this laboratory, like in all labs, keeping the balance of substances prevents any bad eruptions or explosions. The body's "cleansing lab" uses the liver, lungs, skin, colon, kidneys, and all the other parts of your body to flush away the toxins. What is really fascinating is that recent research on genes has revealed a lot of detailed information on the cleaning and protecting abilities of the body.

Toxins and You

How does this magical stuff work in the body's chemistry laboratory? Recent research on genes has proved that the foods you eat "talk" to your genes, bringing them constant information to maintain your health. Scientific research says that your genes get the word from crucial ingredients in foods that activate normal healthy functions, or else the genes get other "words" that give it abnormal instructions. The research has shown that phytonutrients in foods activate the parts of the genes that make detoxification and antioxidant substances to fight off and prevent the toxin "monsters" from taking hold. And at the same time, they shut down the genes that have potential for damaging the body.

FACT

Recent scientific research following the Human Genome Project suggests that diet and environment, more so than your genes, affect your health, longevity, and susceptibility to disease. Current research indicates that some genes that point to the body's greater potential to have a condition or illness are turned "on" or "off" by the foods that you eat.

Toxins are what you want to avoid, but according to researchers the typical American diet and the environment call on the immune system to act frequently. You might imagine that in a continuous red alert the immune system can at times cause a "friendly fire" situation of casualties that can lead to damage in the body. So, is there a way to help the body's cleansing process? Can you cleanse out extra weight, mood swings, aches and pains, poor digestion, "old age" breakouts, and fatigue? Yes, you can, by performing a cleanse.

Types of Cleanses

If the body has a wonderful internal cleansing mechanism, you may wonder why you often have to deal with aches and pains, flus, colds, exhaustion, anxiety, bloat, fat, cloudy brain, and all kinds of things that make the day not so great. A lot of this is due to too many toxins getting into your body, so much so that even the body's miraculous systems can't handle it all alone. It would be great if toxins could be washed off and out of the body so they stop getting in the way of your body's own remarkable cleansing machinery.

There actually are many popular methods and techniques called *cleanses* that are used as a way to detox, recharge, or rejuvenate, or as a jump-start to a healthier life, and hopefully one free of toxins and free radicals. There are scores of reported successes by individuals who have used various cleanse programs. These successes include quick weight loss, better energy, clearer skin conditions, better digestive regularity and processes, clearer mental functioning, better concentration, improved energy and stamina, and better general disposition. Many respected health professionals, as well, agree that certain cleansing regimens can be beneficial.

On the other hand, there are possible risks in some cleansing diets. According to the American Dietetic Association, some cleansing diets can cause nutritional deficiencies, and that can lead to various negative consequences such as muscle breakdown and a weakened ability to deal with infection and inflammation. As a result it is recommended that cleansing diets be avoided by people with diabetes, kidney disease, or heart problems, and those who are pregnant, since some diets can change levels of potassium, sodium, and blood sugars.

The Flush Type of Cleanse

There are many different names and types of flush cleanses that are described as a means of washing and pushing everything out of your system—sometimes also called a *detox cleanse*, *colonic*, or *colonic irrigation*. Many of these plans use the method of drinking certain liquids only, taking special herbs and powders, and sometimes certain supplements. Other plans also use laxatives or enemas, or both, that will "flush out" the colon. Many of these kinds of cleanses are based on the theory that there is a mucus buildup in the colon from undigested foods that make toxins which cause various health problems, and with a colonic irrigation or cleansing, these toxins can be removed. The theory is not yet proven one way or another scientifically. Sometimes doctors do prescribe a colon cleansing as a special preparation for a medical procedure. However, most do not recommend it for a detoxification, believing that the gastrointestinal system works to naturally eliminate bacteria and waste. However, there are many anecdotal reports of individuals experiencing great relief following a reputable colonic.

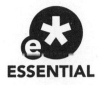

ESSENTIAL

Many health professionals recommend that people interested in a colonic cleanse for a desired relief from a "plugged up" feeling or constipation instead add more fiber-rich foods to their diet, which can have the same, but natural, effect.

Cleansing products that are sometimes used in these cleanses can be labeled "natural," but many health professionals would advise that these products are often not safe, or regulated and tested, and their overall wholesomeness cannot be guaranteed. Health professionals voice concern over these types of cleanses because by inducing diarrhea, they may cause risks of dangerous dehydration, upset the natural balance of colon bacteria, disrupt normal bowel function, and cause potential enema dependence. The intestines are the place where nutrients from food get into the blood and to your body. So, flushing the intestines out in this way may interfere with this process and mean a vitamin or mineral deficiency. Use or continued use of laxatives and products can lead to cramping and bloating, the body falling out of a natural rhythm, and imbalances in electrolytes. Some supplements could interfere with prescription medications that you might be taking.

The Fasting Type of Cleanse

Fasting has been practiced since ancient times. As a spiritual tradition it is still part of rituals practiced today in almost all religions. Many cultures have also used fasting as a means to help people "lighten up" following a winter, and as part of preventive health care. Many medical professionals agree that there is a definite spiritual benefit from fasting, as a part of a spiritual journey, a gateway to mental clarity, self-realization, and as a way to tune into emotions and ideas. However, there are mixed opinions as to the physical benefits of fasting cleanses(also known as simple fasts, modified water or juice fasts, and detox cleanses).

Amy Joy Lanou, PhD, senior nutrition scientist with the Physician's Committee for Responsible Medicine, finds that even though scientific evidence is scarce, the idea of fasting or detoxing makes sense in that by giving the GI cells a rest, because they are not working to avoid toxins, they can potentially become stronger and healthier. She has noted some studies done on fasting that have indicated benefits to people trying to break addictions, and those with chronic conditions.

Joel Fuhrman, MD, a family physician and author of *Eat to Live: The Revolutionary Plan for Fast and Sustained Weight Loss and Fasting and Eating for Health,* has described both negatives and positives of fasting types of cleansing. He does not advise fasting for weight loss since it slows the metabolism. In addition he feels fasting can be dangerous if you have not been maintaining a healthy diet, if you have a compromised immune system, if you are on medication, or if you have liver or kidney problems. On the other hand, he would recommend improving your overall diet and then using a fast as one solution to a buildup of waste products in the cells. "It will only work if you frame the fast with good nutrition before and after. The body is designed to fast; we do it every night," he has said.

Juice fasts can vary in their content and duration but generally are three to five days. Many use a combination of fruit and vegetable juices, usually with added water. The idea is to both alkalinize the digestive system and detox while giving a minimum amount of calories and nutrients. Sometimes the particular fruit or vegetable juices are selected and limited, others more broadly based.

Health professionals would agree that vegetable and fruit juices can be a helpful aid in healing many conditions. Rudolph Ballentine, MD, founder and director of the Center for Holistic Medicine in New York City, voices concerns that people often have low reserves of nutrients because of "empty-calorie" foods, and therefore water fasts can be destructive starvation. However, a regime of a wide variety of vegetable and fruit juices with a supply of basic calories, vitamins, and minerals can guard against protein breakdown and have a cleansing effect.

The Diet Plan Type of Cleanse

There are many different types of diet plan cleanses. Some are designed to target a specific goal such as weight loss; others are plans for a new lifestyle, such as following a diet focused on raw foods or macrobiotics.

While these types of cleanses are called *diet cleanses*, they almost always involve restricting your diet to one or two specific foods that are supposed to achieve the cleanse, and in this ignore the true meaning of the word *diet*—balanced and healthy nutrition.

While weight loss can result from some diet cleanses, there are potential harmful effects. Many times the weight loss is due to fluid and muscle loss. With a large amount of fluid loss there can be headache, dehydration, fatigue, electrolyte imbalance, and mood swings. If calories are very restricted the body's immune system can be weakened, hampering its ability to fight infections, and can cause inflammation. Research has shown that skipping meals and restricting calories slows metabolism, and without enough carbs the body can use muscle for energy. Other side effects can include an inability to focus or concentrate, or a decrease in critical-thinking abilities.

Mixed Method Cleanses

There are also various cleanse programs that use a mixture of flushing, or fasting, and then strict regiments of particular liquids and/or solids, and many times there are prepackaged materials that you must buy from the organization, along with certain supplements that are also provided through purchasing the program. There is as yet no scientific evidence that this method cleanses a body system.

Again, many health professionals caution the use of enemas to cleanse, as they can cause a change in the balance of bacteria in the intestinal tract, which includes a lot of good bacteria.

Some proponents of a slower, three-to-five-day detox diet plan feel it may help motivate a person to make some healthier dietary changes, especially if it is a way to transition to a healthy diet plan. Many health professionals advise to skip the use of enemas, herbal laxatives, saltwater solutions, and such as unproven methods to remove toxins that often are uncomfortable and unpleasant.

The Everything Easy Cleanse

Most recent research on genes has offered news that most illnesses can be prevented and dealt with by the foods you eat. Nutrients are the basis of the best, most healthy cleanse you can give to your body, balancing the intricate chemistry laboratory of the body by putting in nutrients that the typical American diet—made up of mostly foods robbed of these ingredients— takes out. Great nutrients are the best way to help in detox, weight loss, and various bodily issues.

ESSENTIAL

There is no disputing the fact that five servings of fruits and veggies per day is recommended for improving and maintaining overall good health. But very few people have the time or the lifestyle that permits five individual servings in a day. Soup or vegetable juice are great ways to get five servings in a single glass or bowl. A twelve-week study conducted by the University of California found that individuals could make the minimum requirements by drinking just two glasses of vegetable juice per day.

The cleanses suggested and described here are based on offering you great plans and suggestions using as many nutrient-rich meals possible. Food is necessary. Not only do you like to eat, but you also need food to build and repair tissues and to make sure the body keeps its balance and healthy metabolic work so it can most efficiently cleanse. The idea is to follow a plan that balances your nutritional needs and focuses on foods with nutrients that are proven to be crucial for the best-functioning body system. You will boost your body's own natural cleansing ability in a healthy and natural way. Each chapter in this book discusses nutrient-rich foods that benefit particular organs in the body and relate to health issues of that area.

Blending In

These nutrient-rich foods are described, with details about how they work, what they do, and then a cleanse using them is suggested. Recipes are suggested for beverages and soups in blended forms. Why blended beverages and soups, you might ask? Doing your cleanse should not be a difficult, painful experience or a struggle involving starvation. Your cleanse should be an exciting venture—a real present to give to your body and yourself. A present that will set you on your path to a new and healthier you. Research has shown that soups are satisfying! One thing you want your food to do is to satisfy.

FACT

It has been scientifically proven that taking in the same food, with the same nutritional value, is higher in a satiety factor when taken in liquid rather than solid form. Satiety factor is the degree that food or beverage makes you feel full or "satisfied." One such study found that vegetables puréed into a soup or blend had participants feeling fuller and staying fuller longer than the same veggies served on a plate with a glass of water.

Because there are amazing choices, a world of nutrient-rich foods, herbs, and spices that are really important for you and your particular cleanse, the best way to get them in a daily manner is by blending together a few or several of them in a tasty meal—a beverage or soup. In fact, research also has shown that thicker puréed soups, such as in blended soups, offer the best in satisfaction, and for those of you concerned with weight loss, also contributes to that end. People find that after eating blended soup, they are not hungry for a long time afterward. It is often a boon to those who have a problem with snacking and bingeing. And, they can be warm or cold per your preferences.

Nutritious blended soups and beverages are a perfect way to bring a wave of vitamins, minerals, enzymes, and antioxidants that the body needs for efficient cleansing. Also, because they contain a lot of water, blended beverages and soups, along with suggested herbal teas, give the body the hydration that is essential to a cleanse. In many popular cleanses, the idea is flushing out. In this book, the idea is flushing in. Remember the old safety jingle: "in with the good air, out with the bad air"—the same applies to cleansing.

Safety and Realistic Expectations

First and foremost, you should consult with your health professionals to discuss your plans before you undergo any cleanse or diet programs, particularly if you have underlying or chronic health issues.

The cleanses in this book are suggestions that are not carved in stone. They are free and open and easy. Do the best you can with the suggestions, but listen to your bodily needs to feel comfortable, excited, and okay with the process. If you are a coffee drinker, for example, you may wish to modify your amounts. If you are not used to roughage, you may wish to lessen amounts of flaxseed and go gradually with vegetables and fruits, using more of the legumes and whole-grain suggestions.

ALERT

If at any point you feel that your body is not getting what it needs, cease your cleanse *right away and go see a doctor*. Your cleanse should *not* make you feel dizzy, nauseous, faint, weak, or intensely ravenous, and if you feel this way, stop cleansing and adjust your diet plan—you may be trying to do too much! Many people who do cleanses without listening to their body can put themselves in serious health jeopardy.

Cleansing may not be recommended for individuals with chronic infections, those recovering from major surgery, pregnant women, and people with certain diagnosed diseases—physical and emotional—or if you are under doctor's care for any condition. If you fall into any of these categories, please consult with your doctor before entering a cleanse program.

Since the *Everything® Easy Cleanse* idea does not suggest any enemas, laxatives, capsules, supplements, or products that are designed to force the colon to loose its contents, the possible dangers that start with those products are not possible. It is a cleanse plan that suggests healthy fiber, pre- and probiotics, water, and liquids, which is what the colon needs for excellent cleansing. If you suffer from constipation problems, this is the route for you. If you are not used to fiber, go slow with gradual increments to accustom your system to what it needs.

Great Expectations

Just as you can never see your fingernails grow overnight, you may not be able to notice the great work you do with a healthy nutrient cleanse. But keep paying attention to your systems, and systems really will begin to speak to you *with* their satisfactions.

FACT

> Inflammation is part of the body's immune response. Inflammation can lead to anything from joint pain to heart disease. The immune response that causes inflammation is usually triggered by invading bacteria—but not always. Current research suggest that the chemicals in the highly processed foods typical of the American diet can put the immune system into a state of high alert, triggering almost the same kind of inflammatory response as an invading bacteria.

If you are doing a cleanse to lose weight, don't get frustrated when the pounds don't magically melt off after the first week. Don't get agitated when your skin doesn't clear up overnight. Don't quit when you still get headaches after a few days. A cleanse is not a cure-all, but rather a jumping-off point for you on your quest to become a healthier you. If you approach your cleanse as a quick fix, you are setting yourself up for a big disappointment. Cleanses that promise instant results are not reliable, and they are not safe for your body. Besides, a lot of times those cleansers fall right back into their old habits when the cleanse is over, and go back to their old problems.

Set small goals for yourself, like, "Today I'll start a cleanse that will clean out my body's system and make it much easier for me to lose that extra weight," rather than, "I'm going to do this cleanse and look like a million dollars by Friday!" Go into your cleanse with the attitude of someone starting a great journey, and doing something good for yourself to get on the track to better health, and on the track to meet your health and fitness goals in a safe way.

What a Cleanse Is Not

A healthy nutrient cleanse is not a one-time, flush-it-out quick fix. It is a commitment to cleansing not only your body but also your lifestyle, of the physical, nutritional, and even emotional stressors that are negatively impacting your health.

ESSENTIAL

Sally Scroggs, health education manager with the Cancer Prevention Center, says that research is still unclear as to whether or not the cancer-fighting benefits found in herbs, minerals, and other plant compounds are received when taken in capsules, pill, or liquid supplements. Scroggs says that a supplement pill can never replace a healthy diet. She suggests eating a lot of foods packed with cancer-fighting nutrients such as vitamins A, C, and E, betacarotene, resveratrol, selenium, and lycopene.

A cleanse is a jump-start to a healthier lifestyle and wiser food choices. It's not the answer to your prayers or the overnight fix you need to be free of your health problems. If becoming healthy were as easy as cleansing, don't you think a lot more people would be chugging kale smoothies and looking like supermodels? All joking aside, to have a quick-fix view of cleansing is not only wrong, it can also be downright dangerous to your health.

The cleanses presented here are meant to be used for no longer than three days. A cleanse is not a new diet plan that you can use forever, but just the beginning of your new, healthier diet and lifestyle. To continue a cleanse for longer than the recommended amount of time is not good for your body and can even *reverse* the benefits that you are after.

What a Cleanse Is

A true cleanse is like a special kind of vacation from any kind of treadmill of life that's hard to get off. It's a time for you to bring a new kind of healthy comfort to yourself. Doing a cleanse is a time for your body to leave behind some unhealthy habits or traditions and get new ones—as if you are plant-ing seeds of a new, healthy garden inside your body.

The body's natural cleansing machinery is made up of several systems that work together: the liver, the kidneys, the colon, the lungs, and the skin. In some way, shape, or form all of these organs are involved in the processing of nutrients and the elimination of wastes and tox-ins. The better you treat them with good nutrients, the better they will be able to do their jobs of cleansing the body.

A cleanse is an opportunity to do something for just a short period of time that puts you and your body on the path to a healthier, more glowing, more energetic, more alive life!

CHAPTER 2

Cleansing for General Detox

Landscaping makes the world around you look attractive. People also pride themselves on their personal landscapes— their choice of dress, mannerisms, and style. But all that you are on the outside is also affecting your inside! All that you experience, every day, goes inside your body and works to make and shape your life. The outside world is filled not only with beautiful flowers and trees, but its share of garbage as well. Fumes from carpeting, glue, paint, cleaning products, air-conditioning units, lotions, moisturizers, sunscreens, cosmetics, soap, shampoo, deodorants, and antiperspirants are all around you.

Is Your Body a Toxic Waste Dump?

Humans take in toxins everywhere. You experience vision toxins from the images you see—negative, ugly, and disturbing images have an impact on the body and its reactions. Sound toxins, of unnatural frequencies, can throw off the natural balance of the body. The electromagnetic field around the body from satellites, radar, and technology affects your inside as well as your outside.

ALERT

Secondhand smoke contains thousands of toxic chemicals, including: benzene, carbon monoxide, chromium, cyanide, formaldehyde, and lead. Evidence of the health hazards of exposures to secondhand smoke continues to grow. Recent studies have shown that even low-level secondhand smoke exposure during pregnancy can affect fetal growth.

The foods you eat look appetizing, colorful, and smell divine—and much of that is just artificial flavors, coloring agents, additions, emulsifiers, preservatives, flavor enhancers, and reconstitutions, many of which are toxins.

Toxins come into your body at the rate of almost every breath you take in, and your makeup is miraculously designed to deal with them and eliminate the poisons from your body. But your body can suffer overload or have trouble doing its miracle jobs and then it can suffer a breakdown from mild to severe. Depression, anxiety, irritability, sleep problems, aggression, and many cancers have all been linked to toxins in the body.

Typical Body Toxin Issues

Everyday toxins known to be hazardous to your health are released into the air you breathe, the water you drink, and the food you eat. You probably have been ingesting these chemicals and other compounds for years. Many times you cannot see, feel, or even smell toxins in your environment, and you won't even feel their effects until you come down with a chronic condition after years of exposure.

A recent report by the Columbia University School of Public Health estimated that 95 percent of all cancers in the United States are the result of toxicity in diet and the environment. Besides this incredible increased risk of cancer, environmental toxins have been linked to many other conditions from neurological disorders such as Alzheimer's disease to chronic fatigue syndrome. The Collaborative on Health and the Environment has a database on their website (*www.healthandenvironment.org*) that lists 180 separate diseases and conditions that are related to exposure to specific environmental toxins.

ALERT

Dangerous levels of lead are present in the air, soil, and water. Even relatively low levels of lead exposure can be detrimental to brain function in children. And it is not only kids and developing fetuses that have health problems related to lead toxicity. Adults can suffer increased blood pressure and damage to the kidneys, brain, and nervous system, all from exposure to lead.

Following is a list by Dr. Joseph Mercola, a leader in the U.S. wellness movement, of some common toxic substances in the environment, their sources, and conditions exposure to them can cause. It certainly makes one feel unhealthy just to read these and think about them inside of your body:

- **PCBs (polychlorinated biphenyl):** The use of PCBs has been banned in the United States. That is the good news; the bad news is that because it was used for decades it is still a very widespread toxin in our environment.

  Health risks: Cancer, impaired fetal brain development

  Major source: You might be surprised that a very common source of PCBs is farm-raised fish. Most farm-raised salmon are fed pellets made of ground-up fish that have absorbed PCBs and high levels of the chemical are then taken up by the salmon.

- **Pesticides:** According to the Environmental Protection Agency (EPA), 60 percent of all herbicides and 30 percent of all insecticides are known to be carcinogenic. There are some figures that estimate traces of pesticides in as much as 95 percent of U.S. foods.

  Health risks: (other than cancer) Parkinson's disease, nerve damage, miscarriages, and birth defects

  Major sources: Food, especially fruits, vegetables, and commercially raised meats, water (even bottled water!), and bug sprays

- **Mold and other fungal toxins:** Over 30 percent of the population has allergic reactions to mold. Mycotoxins or fungal toxins can cause a range of health problems in sensitive people even in very small amounts. Molds and fungus may not be obvious around a household—even the cleanest of spaces can harbor them.

  Health risks: Cancer, diabetes, asthma, heart disease, multiple sclerosis, dementia

  Major sources: Residential contamination, and foods such as peanuts, wheat, corn, and alcoholic beverages

- **Phthalates:** Chemicals that are used to lengthen the life of fragrances and make plastics stronger and more flexible. Phthalates are like chemical hormones that you may not want in your body.

  Health risks: Endocrine system damages

  Major sources: Plastics—primarily plastic wraps, plastic soda and water bottles, and plastic food storage containers

- **VOCs (volatile organic compounds):** VOCs are one of the large contributors to global warming and depletion of the ozone layer, and are serious health risks.

Health risks: Cancer, visual disorders, respiratory distress, and memory impairment

Major sources: Indoor air, drinking water, and household products such as deodorants, cleaning fluids, and air fresheners

- **Dioxins:** These are results of processes such as commercial or municipal waste incineration and from burning fuels.

  Health risks: Cancer, damage to the reproductive system, skin disorders such as rashes, discoloration, excessive growth of body hair, and mild liver damage

  Major sources: Dioxin gets stored in animal fat, and it is estimated that 95 percent of the beef in the United States is contaminated with dioxins

- **Asbestos:** This is a general name for several forms of the mineral magnesium silicate. It has been used in industry for fireproofing, electrical insulation, building materials, and numerous other purposes. They are all fireproof, in different ways—some can repel heat, others absorb heat.

  Health risks: Mesothelioma (a form of cancer), scarring of the lung tissue

  Major sources: Asbestos was used as insulation from the 1950s to 1970s. When the material becomes old and crumbly it releases fibers into the air that can get breathed in.

- **Heavy metals:** Metals, especially lead, arsenic, and mercury, are found all over the environment and can build up in the soft tissues of your body.

  Health risks: Cancer, Alzheimer's disease, head pain, cognitive difficulties, fatigue, neurological disorders, and decreased production of red and white blood cells

  Major sources: Pelagic fish, drinking water, pesticides, preserved wood and building materials, and dental work

- **Chlorine:** Chlorine is a natural element. It is a yellow-green gas at room temperature. Under the correct pressure and temperature, it can be changed into liquid—as in the common household bleach, and in the disinfectant used in swimming pools.

  Health risks: Eye and skin irritations, asthma, and respiratory distress

  Major sources: Household cleaners and drinking water in small amounts

Best Nutrients That Avoid and Eliminate Toxins

Now that you understand how these toxins get into your body, and why it is so important to good health to get rid of these damaging compounds, how then does eating or drinking certain foods eliminate them? When you hear the word *cleanse* you may think that they are merely "washed" out like rinsing the grounds out of your coffee cup every morning. That may be the effect, but it's not so simple. Nutritional cleansing is more like sending in a posse of cowboys to round up the "bad guys" and bring 'em in. The cleansing nutrients, usually amino acids, found in the "detox" foods actually bind to the toxins on a molecular level within the liver, the body's organ most responsible for removing toxins, forming new compounds that are then excreted.

FACT

Get to know your onions! Onions contain a powerful flavonoid known as quercitin. Quercitin has been shown in lab tests to retard the growth of breast cancer cells. Onions also contain sulfur compounds that aid the liver in detoxification.

Glutathione, pronounced "Gloota-thigh-own," also known as GSH complex, is one of the most important of these "detox sheriffs." It is a powerful antioxidant, made up of three essential amino acids: glycine, glutamic acid, and cysteine. GSH not only plays a major role in cleansing the body of toxins, but it is also essential to cellular health. Studies have shown that if the level of GSH in cells is less than 70 percent, cellular death, which can lead to disease states, can occur.

Cells make their own GSH. But the availability of cysteine can limit GSH. Your body does produce cysteine, but the ability to do so decreases as you get older. This is just the time when you need it most—not only to combat the effects of aging, but also to help rid your body of the toxins that you have been exposed to over the years. To make up for the shortfall, you need to take in foods rich in GSH and cysteine. It is as if your body's GSH, which is already at decreased levels, is being called to do battle on many different fronts—so it's time to send in the cavalry!

ESSENTIAL

Garlic has many healing and detoxifying properties—but if you love to cook with garlic, cut it finely and cook it quickly. When a garlic clove is cut it releases an enzyme called *allicin*. Allicin has been found in several clinical trials to have many medicinal effects. But it does not occur naturally in garlic; it is released when the clove is damaged as a defense mechanism, so the more you cut up the clove, the more it is released. But it degrades quickly and is sensitive to heat.

GSH is, of course, found in abundance in the liver, the body's "Ground Zero" in the war on toxicity. But it is also found in the lining of the lungs to combat toxins in the air, and is essential to providing energy for proper heart health.

GSH enlists other agents for its support: the amino acids glycine and glutamine. Additionally, vitamin B_2 (riboflavin) can help to recycle used-up GSH. Foods high in GHS, cysteine, glycine, and vitamin B_2 are a great way to support your body's "troops" and to help eliminate toxic waste.

What to Put in Your Shopping Cart

When you are getting ready for your cleanse and a more sensible diet, you need to know which foods contain the nutrients you need. This list is not conclusive, but the foods contained herein are great examples of the types of food you should be selecting:

- Some of the best choices for foods high in glutathione are walnuts, asparagus, avocado, broccoli, okra, zucchini, spinach, watermelon, grapefruit, strawberries, orange, tomato, cantaloupe, and peaches.
- For your cysteine choose yogurt, wheat germ, oat flakes, garlic, onion, broccoli, and Brussels sprouts.
- For your glutamine select fish, eggs, beans, cabbage, and beets.
- For glycine inclusion choose sesame seeds, sunflower seeds, and legumes.
- Whey is a rich source of cysteine, glycine, and glutamine.
- Nutritional yeast (but not brewer's yeast—be careful to make that distinction in your purchase) is a wonderful source of B vitamins that are important in liver detox.
- Milk thistle, great for tea, is known as the milk thistle liver detox, which offers major defense against free radicals.
- Cinnamon works to restore healthy levels of GSH.
- The photochemical in parsley is useful as a protector from the carcinogens found in tobacco. There is evidence it also helps in controlling tumor growth.

FACT

Fasting or ritual cleansing is prevalent across many cultures in the anthropological record. Fasting is used for preventive care in Traditional Chinese Medicine (TCM). In many ancient cultures, especially those in northern climates, fasting was used as a way for people to "lighten up" after a long winter and to shed extra fat that was put on to provide added warmth.

How a Cleanse Can Help

Cleansing is something you do all the time—not just showers or baths, but automatic—sweating, sneezing, eliminating. You're always trying to rid yourself of waste, garbage, and pollutants without even thinking. Sometimes you feel polluted . . . and other times in this busy world, you just accept your tiredness, sluggishness, or general lack of energy, as "just the way it has to be."

It becomes easy to either complain about a physical pain or discomfort, or ignore it and worry about it "tomorrow." Meanwhile, the liver, a major center of detox, is working away thanklessly in this world of overwhelming exposure to chemicals and toxins.

ESSENTIAL

Did you know that a great way to detox is to eat "living foods?" Living foods are sprouted greens—such as alfalfa, mung beans, buckwheat, sunflower, and other kinds of sprouted greens. Within these "living foods" vitamins and enzymes, and other vital nutrients, are far more concentrated when the plant is in its sprouted form.

But now that you're thinking about the dump *inside* you, a detox cleanse is a way for you to concentrate on the nutrition that helps the liver's ability to *dump* the garbage out of you!

Many people know too well that "toxic" overstuffed, sluggish, drained, collapsing state following overstuffing the belly at a Thanksgiving meal with all the trimmings. The stomach, a relatively small organ of fist size, is stretched and compromised beyond it's normal capacity, taxed to work harder, and the body may not be able to even move out of the chair! Just think about how good you feel after you finally get rid of all that food—the lightness, the renewal, the *relief*—and you will have an idea of what a good cleanse can do for you! Choosing a cleanse for general body toxins can similarly offer an anyday feeling of relief, lightness, renewal. Just remember that there are many, many wonderful and nutritious foods you can choose from that will help to keep your body cleansed—today, and every day. Using a wide variety of foods in your everyday diet is the way to take the best and the most of what the earth has to offer you for food.

The Detox Cleanse Process

Aim to choose the toxic cleanse for one to three days. Plan to use your fluids, drinks, soups, and teas every hour or half-hour if needed.

Upon rising, drink a large glass of warm water with a squeeze of lemon juice and 1 teaspoon ground flaxseed if you have a tendency to flatulence, or up to 1 tablespoon. These tiny seeds are a powerhouse for omega-3 essential fatty acids, fiber, and phytonutrients. Flaxseed includes a number of vitamins and minerals, including manganese, vitamin B_6, magnesium, phosphorus, and copper. Choose a fruit-based blended drink for the morning and green drinks or soups for lunch and dinner. Snacks in between breakfast and lunch include herbal caffeine-free teas, especially ginger or cinnamon, or a glass of soy/rice/almond milk recipe. Before bedtime have a glass of water with 1 teaspoon to 1 tablespoon flaxseed. Some recipes are suggested at the end of this chapter.

FACT

The Latin or scientific name for flaxseeds is *Linum usitatissimum*, which literally means "most useful." It seems taxonomists knew what they were doing when they named this versatile and highly nutritious little seed.

After the Cleanse

First, congratulate yourself and your body for the detoxifying work it does for you, constantly, and for being a good friend to your body's detox systems. As the old saying goes, "It's a dirty job, but someone's got to do it!" Yes, sometimes, your detox system might be subject to some whims or fancies at a barbecue or party, or a night in a smoke-filled room, but now you'll know how to clean house. But, don't wait until you indulge—anytime at all, any day at all, you know what to look for in your food choices, and what they can do for your body.

You may wish to keep a journal of problem health areas or spots (and realize all the ones that you are thankfully safe from). When you consider the plusses and minuses of your own detox system, you may wish to do another detox cleanse, or look into addressing another specific body area or problem with another cleanse. So, you've accomplished a good pattern if you:

1. Considered all the toxins you want to wash away.
2. Looked a bit more carefully at labels and ingredients of food products.

3. Shared your knowledge—because now you are in the know—about luncheon meats, or checked yourself before giving a child a bright red lollipop that colors the tongue.
4. Are willing and interested in trying new tastes and reacquainting yourself with the real tastes of some foods that had been buried underneath sauces and breading.
5. Remember that food and drink are pleasures, comforts, and now you know about what you can expect them to do in your body.
6. Developed a scale in your mind that tells you about amounts you are consuming.
7. Know how to keep your hard work moving forward. You may repeat this process, now with your firsthand experience. Or, add an additional day or two if necessary.

Following your cleanse, here are some things to keep in mind:

- Keep your drinking/flushing habits alive with herbal teas and water. Mint and peppermint are helpful to aid digestion, chamomile to help reduce anxiety, cinnamon for blood sugar regulation.
- The recommended ratio of carbs, protein, and fats is generally: carbs to about 40–50 percent of your diet, add 25–35 percent protein, and 20–30 percent healthy fats (from nuts, olive, and flaxseed oils, etc.). Fiber is recommended at 25 grams, and sodium under 2,500 mg.
- Always make sure your system has important probiotics and prebiotics. Dairy sources include yogurt, kefir, and cottage cheese. Nondairy sources include tofu, soy yogurt, miso, tempe, and sauerkraut. A great soup that includes your detox nutrients but restores some healthy priobiotics in your system is the walnut soup (see recipes that follow).
- Do some exercise—both cardio and strength training. Aim for four times a week, and walk every day.
- Stretching is important. It increases oxygen and blood flow, and decreases stress.

Gorgeously Green Libation

A lovely, delicious concoction that combines leafy greens, sprouts, and cinnamon to kick off your detox—and it tastes great!

INGREDIENTS | YIELDS 2 CUPS

1 avocado

¼ onion

½ red or green pepper

1 cucumber

1 bunch raw spinach

1 bunch alfalfa sprouts

1 sprig parsley

½ clove of garlic

2 tablespoons toasted wheat germ

¼ cup ground walnuts, almonds, or cashews (soaked in water to soften)

Juice of 1 lemon or lime

½ cup yeast-free vegetable bouillon

1 cup water

Cinnamon, to taste

1. For a cool blender juice, combine all ingredients except bouillon in a blender and blend until smooth.

2. For a warm soup, add ½ cup yeast-free vegetable bouillon and warm (not boil) to taste for soup.

3. For 1–3 days, you may choose to use this soup anytime, as needed.

Best of Broccoli Soup

This soup takes broccoli florets and other detoxing veggies and combines them for a yummy soup that you can have hot or cold.

INGREDIENTS | YIELDS 2 CUPS

1 cup broccoli florets
½ avocado
⅓ cup onion
1 stalk celery
1 handful spinach or kale
1 clove garlic
½-inch ginger
1 tablespoon ground sesame seeds
⅓ cup ground sunflower seeds
1 cup water
½ cup fat-free, plain Greek-style yogurt

For a cool blender drink, place all ingredients, except yogurt, in a blender and blend until smooth. Swirl in yogurt right before serving. For a warm soup, place all ingredients except yogurt in a pan and heat just to warm. Then swirl in yogurt.

Beautiful Beet Beverage

*With carrots, cucumbers, apples, and cinnamon as part of
this recipe, this tasty cleanser can't be "beet!"*

INGREDIENTS | YIELDS 1 SERVING

1 large beet, grated

2 carrots, grated

1 cucumber

¼ cup chopped raw cabbage

1 red apple, cored and chopped

1 cup water

Cinnamon, to taste

Fresh basil, to taste

½ cup nonfat, plain Greek-style yogurt

Grate and chop all your vegetables to make blending easier. Combine all ingredients in blender and blend until smooth.

Double-A Amazing Soup

*Long believed to be a cancer-fighter, this cleanse contains
flax, a seed that you can find in your local supermarket.*

INGREDIENTS | YIELDS 2 CUPS

1 cup asparagus tips

1 avocado

1 clove garlic

½ red bell pepper

¼ cup spinach

2 tablespoons onion

1 tablespoon lemon or lime juice

1 tablespoon flax oil or ground flaxseeds

½ cup tofu

Cayenne pepper, to taste

1 cup water

1. Process or blend in a blender all ingredients until smooth.

2. Add water to desired thickness.

3. If you prefer the soup warm, heat it slightly, just until it feels warm to the back of your hand, but also can be served cold.

Saving Grace Taste

This recipe takes your everyday cup of almond or soy milk
and dresses it up with some detoxing spice!

INGREDIENTS | YIELDS 1 CUP

1 teaspoon ground cinnamon

1 teaspoon ground nutmeg

1 teaspoon ground cardamom

1 teaspoon ground cloves

1 cup almond or soy milk

1. Mix the spices together in a small bowl.

2. Add spice mix to the milk to taste.

3. In a blender, blend the mixture well and serve immediately.

The Excellent Eight

Leafy greens like spinach are great for a liver and general body detox, and this recipe makes good use of it.

INGREDIENTS | YIELDS 2 CUPS

3 tomatoes
1 cucumber
2 green onions with the white portion
½ green or red bell pepper
1 carrot
1 stalk celery
½ bunch spinach
½ bunch parsley
Lemon juice, to taste
1½ cups water
Fresh chopped herbs of choice, to taste

1. Place all the vegetables in a blender and blend together until smooth.

2. Add the lemon juice, water, and herbs, and blend to combine until it is smooth.

3. Serve immediately.

Walnut Winner Cleanser

*They don't call walnuts "brain food" just because they
look like brains; they are a valuable source of omega-3s.*

INGREDIENTS | YIELDS 2½ CUPS

1 cup spinach

1 celery stalk

1 apple, seeded

Juice of 1 lemon or lime

1½ cups water

½ cup walnuts

½ cup nonfat, plain Greek-style yogurt

1. Take the walnuts and grind them very fine in a coffee grinder or blender.

2. Combine the other ingredients except the yogurt and walnuts in a blender and blend until smooth. Then add the ground walnuts and blend to combine.

3. Once the walnuts have been blended into the mixture, swirl in the yogurt and serve immediately.

Melon Mélange

This sweet treat contains delicious fruits and vegetables like watermelon and strawberries to kick off your detox.

INGREDIENTS | YIELDS 3 CUPS

1 cup watermelon

1 cup cantaloupe

½ cup strawberries

2 tablespoons almond butter

1 cup spinach, romaine, or kale

1 stalk celery

1 cup water

2 tablespoons toasted wheat germ

1–2 dried prunes or dates

1. Add all the ingredients to a blender and blend until smooth.

2. Serve immediately.

CHAPTER 3

Cleansing for Optimal Weight Management

It's hard to get dressed in the morning without at least a glance in the mirror at yourself clothed or unclothed—and then what do you see? Most people are dissatisfied with one body part or another, or feel that an article of clothing could fit better. For many people, the feeling of personal beauty resonates with the weight they carry. And you know that weight is there—or not there—when you walk, sit down, try to play a round of tag with the kids, or bend over to pick up the BlackBerry you dropped. The weight you carry, or do not carry, should allow all these things to happen easily. And that is all up to you.

Best Nutrients for Weight Control

Believe it or not, you do not have to starve yourself to lose weight. In fact, you can actually eat quite a bit—but you have to eat the *right* foods. And that means taking in the nutrients that help your body to lose weight by metabolizing fat.

FACT

Traditionally body weight is thought to be a function of the amount of food consumed and calories burned. There is a theory among holistic health practitioners that toxins that have entered the food supply, and therefore your body, are just as responsible, or maybe even more responsible for weight gain, than the amount of food you eat or exercise you get.

There are many weight-loss products that go under the name of GTF, or *glucose tolerance factor*. Researchers are clear that the nutrients, specifically chromium, that go into these "factors" play an important role in blood sugar balance. Other nutrients in GTF are nicotinic acid—a version of vitamin B_3—and the amino acids glutamic acid, cysteine, and glycine—all powerful cleansing and detoxifying nutrients.

Chromium

Of these nutrients, chromium is probably the most active ingredient in GTF. It is believed that chromium improves the ability of insulin to take in glucose. Insulin is the hormone responsible for carrying sugar, or glucose, into the cells where it can be used for energy. After a meal, blood glucose levels begin to rise, and, in response, the pancreas secretes insulin. Insulin's job is to lower blood glucose levels by speeding up the rate at which glucose can get into the cells. It does this by attaching to what is called *receptors* on the outside of cells. Chromium is believed to help or cause the attachment of insulin to those insulin receptors on the cells.

Chromium may also play a role in keeping blood cholesterol levels at a normal level. In addition, chromium is involved in nucleic acid metabolism.

Nucleic acids are the building blocks of DNA, the genetic material found in every cell.

Magnesium

Another essential nutrient for weight loss is magnesium. Several recent studies suggest that the less magnesium in a person's diet, the greater his or her risk for developing diabetes. Again, magnesium is one of those nutrients that helps insulin in its job of processing or removing sugar from the blood, so it is important for keeping normal blood sugar levels.

ESSENTIAL

Eating foods high in magnesium can lower your risk for diabetes. Magnesium-rich foods include nuts, green vegetables, and whole grains. Health experts believe this is because magnesium is a building block for several enzymes that help the body process glucose.

Perhaps just as important to weight loss, and maintaining healthy body weight, magnesium has also been linked to reducing stress. The body has a particular response to stress that is triggered by a hormone called *cortisol*. Stress has been shown to be a major contributor to weight gain, and stress overeating has definitely added to the huge rise in obesity in recent years. Research has shown that magnesium can regulate the levels of cortisol in the body. So, enough magnesium intake can reduce stress.

Theobromine

Another interesting nutrient for weight loss is called *theobromine*. Theobromine is an organic, nitrogen-containing substance that is found naturally in a number of dietary sources, one of which is chocolate! But don't expect to be reading about the M&M's Diet in this or any other book any time soon. Theobromine is a major component of cocoa, and it is only found in nutritive amounts in dark, rich chocolate with a high percentage of cocoa (or *cacao*). It is also found in teas, especially in green tea.

Before you get excited that chocolate can be good for you, and you run for the nearest candy bar, understand that not all chocolate is the same!

To get the cleansing benefits that exist in chocolate it depends on the level of theobromin. The cocoa bean contains about 312mg of theobromine per ounce. Different types of chocolate contain different amounts of theobromine. In general, the darker the chocolate, or the higher the percent of cocoa, the more theobromine it contains. Milk chocolate contains the lowest amounts, and many "milk chocolate" candies today have *no* real cocoa at all, and are just "chocolate flavored."

Theobromine is similar in structure to caffeine, and like caffeine, it belongs to a class of alkaloid molecules found in many plants called *methylxanthines*. Theobromine is an excellent nutrient for weight loss because it has stimulant and diuretic properties similar to caffeine, and has been shown in clinical studies to act as a powerful appetite suppressant, but its stimulating effect is much milder than caffeine's, so it rarely causes those annoying caffeine jitters—or crashes. Theobromine is also the "feel-good" ingredient in chocolate; it stimulates the production of endorphins and can help with depression that often comes with being overweight.

Good Fat, Bad Fat

The process of converting the calories in the food you eat into energy is called *thermogenesis*. This is how calories are "burned." Everything you eat is burned in this way. But there are foods that are considered thermogenic and nonthermogenic. Thermogenic foods increase the thermogenic response, raise metabolism, and cause more calories to be burned.

ALERT

According to the results of a University of Colorado Health Sciences Center study, eating just an extra 40 grams of fat a day can triple the odds of developing diabetes. That is the amount of fat in a typical fast-food burger and side of fries!

Combining foods in certain ways can increase the body's thermogenic response. For example, eating lean proteins with the right amounts of essential fats, dark green vegetables, and whole grains is a great way to pump up the body's fat-burning furnace. Speaking of fat, that is another thing to consider when you think about thermogenesis. Not all fat is created equal.

There is brown adipose tissue (BAT) fat and white fat. White fat is bad fat; it's the stuff you see loaded on the body when it is overweight. Modern science has discovered that BAT is contained in small amounts throughout the body. Its only function is to produce heat, like thermal underwear on a cold winter day; in fact, it is the fat that keeps hibernating animals alive.

ALERT

Thermogenic-inducing foods are great to burn calories and raise metabolism—however, they can be rough on the digestive system. It's a good idea to take a fiber supplement if you are on a high-protein diet, just to keep everything, including your bowels, "moving" toward your goal!

Now, take that hibernating image and think of the foods you eat. Thermogenesis occurs following meals when the body is busy metabolizing the food. The right foods and the right conditions keep BAT and white fat balanced in the body. The problem occurs when you don't eat the right foods or live under the right conditions that allow for a proper BAT/white balance. Most people eat highly processed foods loaded with fats and sugars that the body doesn't have to work hard to metabolize. Add to that a sedentary lifestyle that doesn't move your body enough to fuel your inner furnace, and that is a recipe for obesity. With all that processing in foods, half of the work of digestion is done for you—so it's no wonder people have become so fat and lazy!

Foods with Thermogenic Effects

Hot spices like cayenne, chili pepper, mustard, turmeric, and cider vinegar also have been shown to increase thermogenic effects. Green tea has many health benefits, and it too has been identified as "thermogenic food." A University of Geneva study concluded that "green tea has thermogenic properties and promotes fat oxidation beyond that can be explained by its caffeine content." Before this study, it was believed that the caffeine in green tea was the main cause of weight loss. Now it is known that green tea has thermogenic attributes that make it perfect to use for weight loss.

Bodybuilders have known for years that if you want to reduce fat and build lean muscle mass, you need to chow down on foods high in protein. Many studies are proving them right. Even if you do not want to be the next Mr. or Mrs. Universe, high protein and low carbs are the way to go. One particular study, reported in the *Journal of Nutrition*, concluded that a high-protein diet combined with exercise enhanced weight loss and reduced levels of fats and lipids in the blood. Recent research also indicates that protein-rich foods have a high satiety factor, meaning they curb your appetite, so you stay fuller longer and eat less.

Fiber

No discussion about cleansing nutrients and weight loss could be complete without talking about fiber. Most people know that fiber is nature's great cleanser, but why exactly is the health and fitness world so high on fiber? There are two main types of fiber: soluble and insoluble. Insoluble fiber does not dissolve in water. It binds to water and distends in the intestinal tract, cleanses the colon, and "keeps thing moving." Soluble fiber is the kind of fiber that does dissolve in water; in fact it actually absorbs water. Once you eat it, the body turns it into a kind of thick, gooey gel, which moves very slowly through your body. While that sounds kind of gross, it is actually a good thing. Soluble fiber fills you up and keeps you feeling fuller longer—so you eat less.

FACT

A good breakfast is key to weight loss and any diet plan, but did you know that a better breakfast choice than oats for many people may be barley? Recent studies have shown that barley is significantly more effective than oats in lowering both the body's insulin and glucose responses. Researchers believe that the difference is barley's soluble fiber content, which is four times greater than that of oats.

Fiber also lowers cholesterol, makes protein more digestible, and helps to stabilize insulin. Fiber also is what is called an *indigestible nutrient*. It makes your body work overtime trying to digest it, raising metabolism.

FACT

Many societies throughout the ages have recognized the abilities of plants and foods to control blood sugar. Raw onions, garlic, and mushrooms were used as a diabetes remedy in Europe, ginseng in China, a bread made from barley was used in ancient Persia, cabbage lettuce, turnips, beans, juniper berries, alfalfa, and coriander in many Asian and East Asian cultures. Modern clinical studies have confirmed the ability of all of these foods to lower blood sugar and/or stimulate the production of insulin.

What to Put in Your Shopping Cart

Here are lists of some of the foods that have the important nutrients that will help your body with this cleansing process. Choose as many as you would like for your recipes and your daily diet even after your cleanse.

- **Fiber foods:** spinach, collard greens, cruciferous veggies such as Brussels sprouts, broccoli, cabbage, legumes, oats, soybeans, parsnips, turnip, onions, bran, oat bran, and fruit
- **Protein foods:** fish, lean chicken, eggs (egg beaters, egg whites), whey protein, unsweetened soy protein powder, tofu, fat-free cottage cheese, plain nonfat yogurt, nuts, seeds, unsweetened soy milk, and skim milk
- **Foods with loads of vitamins and minerals essential to weight control:** parsnips, turnips, parsley, garlic, onion, barley, lettuce, cucumbers, celery, beets, tomatoes, leafy greens, fruits, broccoli, cauliflower, cabbage, and squash
- **Foods with omega-3 fatty acids:** fish, walnuts, flaxseed, and green leafy vegetables
- **Amino acid–rich foods:** cottage cheese, fish, seafood, meat, poultry, nuts, peanuts, brown rice, lentils, sesame seeds, avocado, tempeh, and wheat germ
- **Vitamin B foods:** spinach, bell peppers, turnip greens, garlic, cauliflower, celery, cabbage, asparagus, mushrooms, broccoli, collard

greens, Brussels sprouts, turmeric, tuna, cod, salmon, snapper, halibut, chicken, calf liver, and turkey breast

- **Magnesium and folate foods:** beans, turmeric, spinach, squash, mustard greens, pumpkin, soybeans, sunflower seeds, flaxseeds, sesame seeds, green beans, cucumbers, celery, kale, black and navy beans, peppermint and molasses
- **Foods with lipoic acid:** broccoli, spinach, collard greens, Swiss chard, calf liver, round steak, and yeast
- **Foods with carnitine:** beef, milk, codfish, chicken, and Cheddar cheese
- **Foods with chromium:** romaine lettuce, onions, tomatoes, brewer's yeast, oysters, liver, whole grains, and bran cereals
- **Beverages:** green tea and unsweetened cocoa powder
- **Herbs and spices:** cayenne, mustard seed, ginger, cinnamon, and chili pepper
- **Sweeteners:** stevia and agave nectar
- **Natural diuretics to eliminate bloating and puffiness:** alfalfa, cucumber, lemon, and melons

According to a Penn State University study, your body recognizes soup as a solid food, rather than a liquid, and therefore even a clear broth soup has a high degree of satiety (feeling full) for its density. The study found that people who drank 10 ounces of water before a meal ate much more at the following meal than the group who had the same 10 ounces of water cooked into a clear broth soup. So have a small bowl of a healthy soup before lunch or dinner, and you will eat less.

How a Cleanse Can Help

Everything today has gotten smaller, lighter, and more compact . . . and maybe that's because most people don't like to carry around any kind of "baggage." Your weight is also a kind of baggage that you carry around needlessly. The cleanse will be a super step to rebalance your body, for a new way to carry the weight you want.

Begin your morning with a large glass of water—about 12–16 ounces with 1–2 teaspoons of ground flaxseed to get your insides moving and flushing. Choose your first cleansing meal from a fruit based/protein recipe. Choose a lunch and a dinner meal. A minimum of every hour, have a beverage of green tea with caffeine, plain or with added spice as you wish, cinnamon or ginger tea, and water. Snack with cocoa, if desired, one time per day. Make sure you don't go longer than one hour before another water or beverage. For an easy broth that you can drink any time, dice a mix of four kinds of veggies—your choice—to make 1 cup worth. Add it to 1 quart of water and simmer 10–15 minutes. Strain it and enjoy the broth.

Aim to do your cleanse for one to three days. Some recipes are suggested here.

ESSENTIAL

Your metabolism does slow down at night even while awake, and even more when you sleep. To lose weight do not eat any big meals after 7 P.M., and especially not right before you go to sleep. Eating a big meal right before bed time is the surest way to pack on some extra pounds, as the slow sleeping metabolism will fail to use the food as energy, and just store it as fat.

Just remember that there are many, many wonderful and nutritious foods you can choose from that will help to keep your body cleansed—today, and every day. Using a wide variety of foods in your everyday diet is the way to make the most of what the earth has to offer.

After the Cleanse

First, congratulate yourself and your body for your teamwork in supporting only the weight you want. Yes, sometimes, you might be subject to some whims or fancies at a barbecue or party, or there's that large popcorn at the movies, but now you'll know how to get back to regulations. Never deny yourself some enjoyment and pleasure from eating—and the appropriate treats. But now you are in better touch with what you need, more in touch with what to look for in your food choices and what they can do for your body—so that the next time you touch that body, you will feel that pride—instead of the jiggle!

ESSENTIAL

A generation ago when most meals were taken at the family dinner table, obesity levels were far lower. Scientists say this is no coincidence. Eating seated at the dinner table, the same time, same place, habituates the body to associate eating, and therefore hunger and appetite, with one place and time. Eating "on the go" can cause overeating. So sit down at the dinner table; it will give you more quality time with your kids, and may help your waistline.

You may wish to create a journal of foods taken from the recommended lists that do well with your metabolism and lifestyle, and those that are not working. This way you'll see evidence of the plusses and minuses of your own menu of foods that are right for your body and weight goals—and that you like to eat. You may wish to do another weight cleanse, or look into addressing another specific body area or problem with another cleanse.

So, you've accomplished a good pattern if you:

1. Considered the changes you want your body to learn, and gave your body an excellent lesson.
2. Looked a bit more carefully at labels and ingredients of food products, and the glycemic counts.
3. Are willing and interested in trying new tastes, and reacquainting yourself with the real tastes of some foods that had been buried underneath sauces and breading.
4. Have retrained you body to feel healthy and want to stay healthy.
5. See food and drink as a pleasure, a comfort, and now you know about what you can expect it to do in your body.
6. Have now developed a scale in your mind that tells you about the amounts you are consuming, feeling it go down and around and out.

Following your cleanse, here are some things to keep in mind:

- Begin to increase your selection and amounts of solid foods. A great interim meal suggestion is to spread 1 slice of whole-grain pita with 1 teaspoon of hummus, and top with a ½ can of mashed sardines and a slice of tomato. Sprinkle with 1–2 teaspoons of flaxseed and fresh herbs to your taste.
- Keep your drinking/flushing habits alive with herbal teas and water. Mint and peppermint are helpful to aid digestion, chamomile to help reduce anxiety, cinnamon for blood sugar regulation.
- Walk every day—wherever you can—life will be a longer, healthier path if you do.
- Stretching is important. It increases oxygen and blood flow, and decreases stress.

Most important, keep your hard work moving forward by:

1. Choosing foods that keep blood sugar levels even. Look for fibrous, low-glycemic carbs and focus on unprocessed carbohydrates. If you must eat higher-glycemic carbs, do try to balance it with the lowest glycemic carbs.
2. Eating six small meals every day. Digestion requires calories to burn, and with smaller frequent meals you keep supplying your body with nutrients while it is working to digest, and can then be raising your metabolism.
3. Keeping your metabolism in an even state by eating a nutritious snack before and after exercise.

Add some weight training to your week—even if it's spending a few minutes with your heavy bag of groceries! Evidence has shown that weight training raises your metabolism. High-cardio aerobic activity also moves your body into processing waste and keeping the metabolism elevated, even after the exercise finishes.

Liquid Protein Power Punch with Strawberries

A delicious fruit as well as a nutritious addition to any meal or snack,
this recipe features the only fruit with the seeds on the outside—a strawberry!

INGREDIENTS | YIELDS 1 SERVING

3 ounces liquid egg whites

2 tablespoons unsweetened whey or soy protein powder

2 teaspoons ground flaxseed

½ cup soy milk or skim milk

5–6 strawberries

2 tablespoons unsweetened toasted wheat germ

Stevia, to taste

1 cup water

2–3 ice cubes (optional)

1. Add all ingredients to the blender and blend until smooth.

2. Drink this mixture as one or all of your daily meals (every few hours) for up to three days.

Liquid Protein Power Punch with Mocha

Who says mocha always has to come in an expensive, calorie-filled coffee treat from a chain store? This recipe uses the power of mocha for health!

INGREDIENTS | YIELDS 1 SERVING

3 ounces liquid egg whites

2 tablespoons unsweetened whey, or soy protein powder

2 teaspoons ground flaxseeds

2 cups soy or skim milk

½ cup coffee

1 tablespoon unsweetened cocoa

¼ teaspoon cinnamon, or to taste

Stevia, to taste

1 cup water

2–3 ice cubes (optional)

1. Combine ingredients in a blender and blend until smooth.

2. Drink this mixture as one or all of your daily meals for up to three days.

Cute and Creamy Cucumber-Cantaloupe Beverage

Fresh fruits are antioxidants and have been proven to help cut cancer risks in half. Strawberries, cantaloupe, and pear are low on the glycemic indexes, so they don't spike weight gain.

INGREDIENTS | YIELDS 1–1½ SERVINGS

½ cucumber

½ cup cantaloupe

½ teaspoon lemon or lime juice

1 cup chopped romaine or kale

1 teaspoon ground flaxseeds

2 tablespoons toasted wheat germ

½ cup fat-free cottage cheese

1–2 dried, pitted prunes

1 cup water

Stevia, to taste

2–3 ice cubes (optional)

1. Combine all ingredients in a blender and blend until smooth. Bigger ingredients like the cantaloupe and fruit may be blended alone first, as they may need more time to blend.

2. Drink this mixture as one or all of your daily meals for up to three days.

Coaxing Cocoa

Cocoa powder not only tastes great, but is also a great way to jump-start a weight loss program. But don't be fooled—chocolate from the store has added sugars and dairy products that make it an unhealthy choice.

INGREDIENTS | YIELDS 1 CUP

2 teaspoons cocoa powder

1 cup hot water

1 teaspoon ground flaxseeds

1 teaspoon ground sunflower seeds

¼ cup unsweetened soy milk or skim milk

1 teaspoon stevia, or to taste (optional)

¼-½ teaspoon cinnamon, or to taste

1. In a small bowl, mix the cocoa powder and hot water together until the powder is dissolved.

2. Place the ground flaxseeds, ground sunflower seeds, and soy milk (along with the cocoa powder mixture) into a blender and blend until smooth.

3. Add the stevia and the cinnamon to your taste.

4. Drink this mixture as one or all of your daily meals for up to three days.

Valuable Veggie Soup

Here's a great nutritious and delicious salad in one bowl.
Flaxseed adds high omega-3 "good" fat content.

INGREDIENTS | YIELDS 2 SERVINGS

1 carrot, chopped or diced

1 celery stalk

1 cucumber

½ cup chopped romaine leaves

¼ cup chopped cabbage

1 tablespoon fresh parsley

¼ cup chopped onion

½ garlic clove

1 teaspoon paprika

¼ cup ground raw sunflower seeds

⅓ cup ground walnuts or cashews
(soaked in water to soften, 1–2 hours for cashews, or overnight for walnuts)

1 tablespoon ground flaxseeds

1 cup water

1. Add the carrots, celery, and cucumber to a blender and blend together.

2. Add the remaining ingredients and blend together until smooth.

3. Drink this mixture for one or all of your daily meals for up to three days.

Asian Activating Soup

This flavorful concoction has savory ingredients like ginger and cilantro that wake up your taste buds and get your body ready to burn some fat.

INGREDIENTS | YIELDS 2 SERVINGS

1 cup water
1 cup cabbage
½ onion
1 carrot
1 red bell pepper, chopped
½ inch gingerroot
1 clove garlic
½ cup mushrooms
¼ cup chopped fresh cilantro
1 tablespoon flaxseeds, or to taste
¼ teaspoon black pepper or red pepper flakes
¼ teaspoon ground star anise
¼ teaspoon ground fennel seeds
¼ teaspoon ground cloves
¼ teaspoon ground cinnamon

1. Add all the ingredients to a blender and blend until smooth.

2. This recipe may be served warm or cold. If you prefer it warm, transfer the mixture from the blender to a pot on the stove. Simmer until warm, when a drop feels warm to the back of your hand.

3. Drink this mixture for one or all of your daily meals for up to three days.

Benefits of Spicy Foods

Studies have shown that spicy foods are a "hot pick" to boost metabolism. Scientists looking at the process of thermogenesis have found that hot, spicy ingredients can cause the metabolism to shoot up by as much as 25 percent. That can translate to burning off forty-five extra calories in just three hours—so the next time you crave that guacamole, leave off the sour cream but don't forget the hot sauce!

Eggcellent Experience Soup

Eggs are an excellent source of protein, especially when they are the primary ingredient in a dish. This recipe features eggs prominently.

INGREDIENTS | YIELDS 1 SERVING

1½ cups fat-free, unsalted broth
2 whole eggs
1 egg white
2 tablespoons cold water
Pinch pepper
Pinch ginger
Pinch cayenne
1 teaspoon ground flaxseeds

1. In a large pot, bring the broth to a boil.

2. While the broth is heating, beat the eggs and egg white with the water, pepper, ginger, cayenne, and flaxseeds.

3. Pour the egg mixture slowly into the broth, while swirling it with a whisk or fork to create a noodle like appearance. When all the egg has become "noodlelike" in the water, in 1–2 minutes, the soup is ready to serve.

Floret Fantastic Fuel

Broccoli is a great source of chromium, a mineral with the ability to regulate blood sugar. One cup of broccoli has been estimated to contain 22 micrograms of chromium, which is about ten times more than any other food.

INGREDIENTS | YIELDS 1–2 SERVINGS

1 cup water

1 cup cauliflower and broccoli florets mixed

1 carrot

3 leaves romaine lettuce

1 clove garlic

2 tablespoons chopped fresh dill

1 tablespoon sesame tahini

1 teaspoon ground flaxseeds if you are new to flaxseeds, or 2 teaspoons to help with constipation difficulties

¼ teaspoon parsley

Ground black pepper, to taste (optional)

½ cup nonfat, plain Greek-style yogurt

1. Combine all ingredients, except the yogurt, in a blender and blend until smooth.

2. Add the yogurt and swirl until desired smoothness.

3. This mixture can be served warm or chilled. If you desire it warmed, transfer the mixture to a pot on the stove and heat until a drop feels warm on the back of your hand.

Celery Soup

Here's a combination of nutrient rich veggies.

INGREDIENTS | YIELDS 1–2 SERVINGS

3 celery stalks, chopped

1 tomato, chopped

1 yellow or red bell pepper, chopped

½ zucchini, chopped

½ cucumber, chopped

1 teaspoon chili powder and/or a dash of cayenne, to taste

1 teaspoon ground flaxseeds

1 clove garlic, chopped

1 tablespoon fresh parsley

1 tablespoon fresh basil

3 leaves romaine lettuce, chopped

1 cup water

½ cup nonfat, plain Greek-style yogurt

1. Combine all ingredients, except the yogurt, in a blender and blend until smooth.

2. When the mixture is at the desired smoothness, add the yogurt and stir until mixed thoroughly.

3. Drink this mixture for one or all of your daily meals for up to three days.

Tofu Toughing It Spicy Protein Soup

Both ancient and modern studies show that onions have the ability to lower blood sugar. Onions are a great aid in metabolism of glucose and release of insulin.

INGREDIENTS | YIELDS 1 SERVING

½–1 clove garlic

½ inch ginger, grated

1 teaspoon chili powder, or to taste

1 teaspoon apple cider vinegar

1 teaspoon lemon or lime juice

1 red or green bell pepper, seeded and chopped

½ cup mushrooms, chopped

½ cup spinach, chopped

1 sprig watercress leaves

2 scallions, or 1 tablespoon chopped onion

½ cup tofu

2 teaspoons ground flaxseeds

1½ cups water or low-sodium broth

1. Combine all ingredients in a blender and blend until smooth.

2. Transfer mixture from blender to pot on the stove. Heat the mixture until warm, when a drop feels warm on the back of your hand.

CHAPTER 4

Cleansing for
Healthy Digestion

What can be worse than eating something that looks beautiful and smells even better, and then ending up with belching, gas, bloating, waist buttons popping, rumblings, and a long time in the bathroom? What can be better than you eating something that delights the senses, looks inspiring, and has an intensity of aromas—and after eating, you feel terrific, energized, clearheaded, without the rumbles, bumbles, or next-day potty blues?

Typical Digestive Issues

The truth is, not all the foods that look appetizing or fun make for pleasant situations in the digestive system. But the good news is that there are many food choices that have been proven with research to be excellent for you and your belly and digestion.

ALERT

Digestion actually begins in the mouth, and one sure way to improve digestion is to slow down, take smaller bites, and chew your food properly. Taking the time to sit down, enjoy, and not rush through meals will reduce stress and help your digestive system. Wolfing down meals and swallowing improperly chewed food makes your digestive system work much harder than it has to.

So, this is the time to get rid of those pain-causing foods—the junk that makes your belly feel like junk. Plan for a way to have a nice, satisfied belly full of food nutrients that are good for you now and for any day.

The "Ins and Outs" of Your Digestive System

It is no coincidence that when something is wrong or "off," people often say they can "feel it in their guts." Many cultures believe that the "gut," or the digestive system, is the key to all heath and well-being. Even the rage in Pilates today is all about centering—needing and using your core, your all-important stomach muscles to keep you upright and energized. Of course, the work of the whole digestive system involves the long process from the time food goes into the mouth, through what happens to get the nutrients out of the food, and then how to get rid of the garbage and wastes. Eating the proper foods is the key to proper digestion.

Digestive issues are common, and just about everyone has experienced one or more at times. The most common issues include stomachaches, nausea, heartburn, gas, constipation, diarrhea, irritable bowel syndrome (IBS), and allergies. Digestive issues can be embarrassing and inconvenient, and worse yet, there is the pain and debilitation.

Sometimes digestive issues pose serious health risks, needing hospitalization, or even ending up in death. It is always wise to seek medical attention for any issue that may be a serious problem.

ESSENTIAL

Not that fond of stewed prunes? Try a stewed apple or pear as tasty accompaniment to a healthy breakfast of warm whole-grain cereal with almonds or cashews, or whole-grain bread spread with almond or cashew butter. Add a little rice, soy, almond, or skim milk and you'll be ready to go.

Digestion really starts in the stomach, and young or old, everyone has had his or her share of tummy aches. Heartburn or indigestion are not really the correct words for the issue for a number of reasons. It got that name *heartburn* because one usually experiences the feelings in the chest. But heartburn has nothing to do with your heart. In fact, it is a stomach issue. The symptoms of heartburn happen when stomach acid backs up into the esophagus, which does not have the same protection from gastric juices that the stomach's lining has. This is also called *gastrointestinal esophageal disease*, or GERD or "acid reflux." One in ten Americans experiences this type of heartburn at least once a week. Heartburn has different triggers in different people. Causes can vary from food sensitivities to being overweight, to stress.

ALERT

Spicy foods can cause heartburn in sensitive individuals, but spices can also aid in digestion in a few ways. Cumin, coriander, mustard, garlic, cinnamon, paprika, cayenne, and black pepper all work to increase salivation, which is the first step of digestion. Spicy foods also cause you to drink more water. Spices in food can also aid digestion by increasing the production of bile, which can help your body break down and absorb fats.

Nausea and vomiting are some other common stomach problems. Nausea can be caused by any number of triggers from food poisoning, to motion sickness, to emotional distress.

FACT

You probably know about aloe vera and skin care, but when juiced and drunk, aloe vera also helps in cleansing of the digestive tract. Try 2 to 3 ounces of aloe vera juice mixed with pure water for a refreshing pick-me-up.

Ulcers are another cause for abdominal upsets. Ulcers are sores in the stomach lining. It was once thought that extra acid was the cause of most stomach ulcers. However, recent research has shown that ulcers are usually caused by the *H. pylori* bacteria.

When You Can't Go

Moving away from the stomach, and further down the gastrointestinal track, there can be more issues. Constipation or irregularity is one of the most common digestive issues. Common irregularity is uncomfortable and stressful. Continuous or chronic constipation can lead to serious health problems. The medical dictionaries say you are constipated if you have less than three bowel movements in a week.

ALERT

A great natural and gentle laxative is ground flaxseeds. To help regularity try sprinkling ground flaxseeds on salads, rice, or into any meal of your choice.

Despite what many people think, there really is no rule that says you need to have a movement every day. Diet and activity level all affect how often a person generally has bowel movements. Your body will tell you what is "regular" for you based on your own system and lifestyle. No matter how being "irregular" is defined for you, whether it has been days or just a few hours, being constipated can make you feel "plugged up," slow, bloated, sluggish, or just plan miserable.

Constipation doesn't always mean not having any movements at all; constipation can also be characterized by small, very solid, and hard-to-pass feces. With constipation there is often stomach cramps. Left untreated, constipation could lead to serious health issues.

When You Can't Stop Going

The opposite side of constipation is diarrhea. Like constipation, diarrhea is not usually a topic for light cocktail party conversation, but also like constipation, the truth is, it is something you have probably had to deal with at one point or another.

Diarrhea can affect anyone at any age. It is medically defined as a watery or loose stool. Doctors break down diarrhea into three categories: osmotic, secretory, and exudative. It is not usually life threatening, except in extreme cases such as when its cause is parasites, food poisoning, or other severe bacterial infection. The biggest danger with diarrhea is dehydration. Most mild cases of diarrhea will clear up in a few days on their own. In fact, other than to keep drinking fluids, many medical practitioners say not to treat diarrhea immediately upon its onset, because diarrhea is part of your body's defense mechanism, and it is one of its ways of getting rid of whatever it is that is making you ill.

It's a Gas

Gas is experienced in two different ways: burping and flatulence, both of which children find rather amusing—adults not so much. Certainly when too much gas is produced, it is no laughing matter for anyone of any age. Too much gas causes pain, bloating, and stomach cramps. Many times the gas is caused by digestion problems in processing certain foods including lactose in milk, grains, and gluten in some carbohydrates. There are some natural remedies that can help with problems of gas. Most important is to eat slowly, chewing your food well. Don't be gulping gobs down the hatch. Peppermint, spearmint, or anise tea after a meal can be helpful. Soak some slices of peeled ginger root in lemon juice, and chew a slice after a meal.

Irritable Bowel Syndrome

While everyone likely suffers from common digestive issues like gas, diarrhea, constipation, and heartburn from time to time, some people can experience any and all of them on a regular basis. They suffer from perhaps the most chronic of digestive issues, irritable bowel syndrome (IBS). Like many digestive issues, the main causes of IBS are not completely and perfectly known.

FACT

Food allergies or sensitivities are responsible for many digestive issues. Over 50 percent of IBS patients report having one or more food intolerances, causing symptoms such as gas, bloating, and pain. The most common foods reported are milk, dairy, and grains.

What is known is that in people with IBS the colon contracts more quickly than in people without IBS. There are many different situations that trigger those contractions and therefore an attack of IBS. Triggers have been found to include: reactions to certain foods, reactions to medications, artificial sweeteners such as sorbitol and malitol, and emotional stress. Just as the triggers of a bout of IBS vary from person to person, so do its symptoms. IBS is often confused with IBD, or inflammatory bowel disease, which is a far more serious issue. IBS does not involve inflammation of the bowel.

Crohn's Disease

Inflammatory bowel disease, also known as Crohn's disease, is a chronic illness in which the intestine becomes inflamed and ulcerated with sores. That is why IBD is also known as ulcerative colitis. Colitis, enteritis, and ileitis are all other forms of Crohn's or IBD. No matter what it is called, it always involves inflammation of the bowel or intestine, and it is a serious medical condition that requires a doctor's care. Current research suggests that Crohn's is an autoimmune disease where the body reacts to its own intestine as if it were foreign tissue. Nutrition and lifestyle changes can be a help to lessen this autoimmune response.

A homemade broth made from vegetables and fish bones can help with more thorough digestion of carbohydrate and protein foods. This type of gelatinous broth has been used effectively for the treatment of many chronic digestive disorders, including Crohn's disease.

Hemorrhoids

Hemorrhoids are very common; almost every adult will have them at some time or another. While uncomfortable, and embarrassing, hemorrhoids are not usually a serious health threat. A hemorrhoid is a bit of swollen tissue that is within the anal canal, the tube that connects the rectum with the anus. The inflamed tissue causes itching and discomfort.

With all digestive issues, prevention is key. Great nutrition and a healthy lifestyle can prevent them from happening and can keep your digestive system happy and healthy.

Tummy ache? Ayurvedic medicine practitioners suggest a fresh piece of ginger sprinkled with lemon juice, or a glass of buttermilk with a pinch of cumin and coriander. Also, a leading cause of constipation is lack of hydration, so make sure you drink a lot of water!

Best Nutrients for Good Bowel Function

In no other system in the body is what you put in more related to "what comes out" than in the digestive system. Eating the right foods is key to not only keeping things moving along, but also to ensure that the nutrients from that food that are absolutely important to all other body systems are used and absorbed correctly.

Test Your Moral "Fiber"

As you might imagine, the most important nutrient to proper digestion is fiber. There are two kinds of fiber, soluble and insoluble, and both are needed to avoid many digestive problems.

Soluble fiber dissolves in water; insoluble fiber does not. Insoluble fiber is the one that most people think about in terms of lending a hand with irregularity, and it is especially helpful in keeping the colon healthy and preventing constipation or difficult bowel movements.

ALERT

Fiber is critical to keeping the "good bacteria/bad bacteria" in the gut in proper balance. Some people cannot tolerate major increases of additional fiber. Add more fiber to your diet gradually by eating fruits and veggies with less roughage at first, such as pears, bananas, applesauce, and well-cooked squash.

Soluble fiber helps the growth of "good" bacteria in the gut, which in turn make natural antibiotics that stop the growth of the "bad" bacteria such as *Salmonella*, *Campylobacter*, and *Escherichia coli* (E. coli). Many scientists and medical professionals believe that high levels of these "good" bacteria in the intestines may also help to prevent colon cancer.

You need about 20 to 35 grams of fiber per day. In today's world of overprocessed foods, few people get more than 10 grams. To meet the fiber requirement, it is important to eat five or more servings of fruits and vegetables and six or more of whole grains every day. But fiber is only part of the story about nutrient-rich foods that can help to keep the bowels clean, healthy, and functioning well.

Enzymes

Enzymes are crucial to correct digestion. Enzymes are proteins that are secreted by all of the organs of the digestive system that help the body break down foods. These enzymes have also been shown to help the growth of healthy bacteria and lessen the growth of harmful flora in the intestines. The digestive system does make these enzymes, known as *proteases*, *peptidases*, and *lipases*, but they are also in some of the foods that you eat. A diet rich in these enzymes can make sure there is a healthy amount of them in the digestive system for them to do their great work.

FACT

A medium-sized avocado has a whopping 15 grams of fiber, making it pound for pound one of the most fiber-rich fruits around. Avocados are very easy on the digestive system and contain plenty of healthy, raw monounsaturated fat.

Lipase is the enzyme that breaks down fat. Lipase is important as it helps to rid the body of triglycerides and cholesterol, and in digestion, lipase is responsible for making it easier for nutrients to be absorbed by cells.

Many of the plant-based enzymes are not made by the human digestive system. But research has evidence that since they help plants to absorb their own nutrients, they can also aid in human digestion. One such enzyme is bromelain, found in pineapples, which helps to break down proteins. Another is betaine HCL, found in beets. Like bromelain, betaine also helps with the breakdown of fats and proteins, and it has the added benefit of helping to relieve bloating, belching, and flatulence. Another, papain, found in papaya, once again is an aid in the breakdown and absorption of proteins, and it also soothes upset stomachs and may help prevent ulcers.

Fiber and enzymes can both be found in the foods you eat, and both help increase healthy bacteria in the digestive system.

Bacteria Can Be Nice

One "friendly bacteria" is *Lactobacillus bifidus*. This bacteria helps to keep a healthy amount of bacteria in the large intestine; it also increases the acidity there, which stops the growth of the more dangerous bacteria.

Related to lactobacillus is the nutrient lactic acid. Not to be confused with *lactose*—a sugar that is the cause of lactose intolerance, which is a digestive problem—lactic acid can actually aid digestion. Lacto-fermented foods, such as kefir, are wonderful sources of the lactic acid that can help digestion. The lactic acid in these foods helps to break down protein and helps in the absorption of iron, calcium, and other nutrients from all foods.

Amino Acids

There are several amino acids, once again found mostly in plants—fruits and vegetables—that help to keep your guts healthy and working normally. Digestion breaks down protein into amino acids so that the body can then use those amino acids as raw materials to build new proteins that the body needs to function. However, there are amino acids that you can eat in food that can help the process. Glutamine is one of these. It is an important amino acid for keeping up the works of the intestine, and it has been shown to repair damage to the mucosal linings of the bowel. Methionine and N-acetyl cysteine are sulfur-containing amino acids that are essential to the production of GSH, a key antioxidant for protecting cells from free-radical damage. GSH helps to keep all bodily systems working at their best, including digestion.

ALERT

Raw plant fats are very helpful to the health of your digestive tract. Raw fats such as those found in avocados, young coconuts, nuts, and raw, cold-pressed oils stimulate healthy work of your gall bladder, pancreas, and liver.

What to Put in Your Shopping Cart

Here are the foods that are high on the important nutrients for your cleanse. Choose as many as you wish now and include them in your daily diet after your cleanse.

- **Fiber foods for digestive health and regularity:** fresh fruits, especially pears and apples, fresh vegetables, all whole grains, nuts, bran, and flaxseeds
- **Whole grains:** brown rice, buckwheat, corn, millet, quinoa, whole wheat, oats, and barley
- **Proteins:** eggs, fish, chicken, lamb, miso, tofu, and tempeh
- **Healthy fats including omega-3s:** olive oil, flaxseed oil, flaxseeds, salmon, walnuts, sardines, halibut, snapper, soybeans, and tofu

- **Foods containing calcium and magnesium:** spinach, broccoli, almonds, kale, beet greens, sunflower seeds, sesame seeds, watercress, parsley, coconut, walnuts, and corn
- **Spices and herbs:** coriander, cumin, mustard, garlic, cinnamon, paprika, cayenne, pepper, ginger, fennel, clove, peppermint, cilantro, basil, rosehips, and aloe
- **Probiotics and prebiotics:** yogurt, kefir, kimchi, tempeh, kombucha, bananas, chicory root, onions, leeks, fruit, soybeans, sweet potatoes, asparagus, and some whole grains

FACT

Some of your best sources of dietary fiber are dried fruits, such as dates, figs, and prunes. Legumes and beans are also a good source. Canned beans are okay for those who do not have time to cook dried beans. Lentils and split peas will leave you less gassy than other legumes.

How a Cleanse Can Help

Belly and bottom issues are usually no joke to the one who has them. Reacquainting your digestive system with the best of nutrients for its best work in a cleanse for digestion, and leaving some of the damaging foods behind, will start you off to a good working relationship with your own body.

Aim to do the digestion cleanse for one to three days. Plan to use your fluids, drinks, soups, and teas every hour or half-hour as needed.

Upon rising, drink a large glass of warm water with a squeeze of lemon juice and 1 teaspoon ground flaxseeds, which is great for constipation. If you don't have a tendency toward flatulence, use up to 1 tablespoon. These tiny seeds are a powerhouse for omega-3 essential fatty acids, fiber, and phytonutrients. Choose fruit-based or vegetable-based blended drinks and soups for breakfast, lunch, and dinner. Some recipes are suggested later in the chapter.

Snacks in between breakfast and lunch include herbal caffeine-free teas or some digestive drink suggestions. Ayurvedic traditions often recommend fennel seed or cumin seed tea for digestion. Boil 1 cup of water, add

1 teaspoon fennel or cumin seed, and a pinch of stevia (if desired), cover, and steep five to twenty minutes. Strain and drink at room temperature.

ESSENTIAL

> Bananas have long been known for their ability to quench stomach acids, give protection from stomach ulcers, and help to relieve the pain of ulcers. There are nutrients in bananas that make the lining of the stomach thicker and stop the growth of bacteria known to cause ulcers. If you have been suffering with a bad case of diarrhea, reach for a banana; they are a great source of potassium, a necessary electrolyte that diarrhea depletes.

A glass of water with ¼ cup of blended watermelon or blended cucumber can also be a boon for constipation problems. A blend of 1 carrot, ½–1 banana, and ½ cup water can also be used.

A suggested snack that is often recommended is a Lassi, a nice yogurt mixture for the belly. Blend ¼–½ cup yogurt, 1 cup water, and a pinch each of ginger, cumin, coriander, and salt.

Before bedtime have a glass of water with 1 teaspoon to 1 tablespoon flaxseed, for constipation issues.

After the Cleanse

First, take a deep breath and congratulate yourself and your body for taking the time to treat your digestive system with loving nutritious concern and care. Your system won't always stay in perfect order, but now you'll know more about your digestive system's own language and what to say to it. Following your cleanse, here are some things to keep in mind:

- Begin to increase your selection and amounts of solid foods. A great interim meal suggestion is to spread a slice of whole-grain pita with 1 teaspoon of hummus, and top with a ½ can of mashed sardines in olive oil or tomato sauce.
- Keep your drinking/flushing habits alive with herbal teas and water. Mint and peppermint have historically been a helpful herbal remedy

to aid digestion, chamomile to help reduce anxiety, cinnamon for blood sugar regulation. A refreshing juice, a holistic recommendation for digestion is a blend of 1 orange or tangerine segments, ¼ papaya, 1 teaspoon ground flaxseeds, 2 teaspoons fresh mint, 2 teaspoons fresh parsley, and 1 cup water.

- Always make sure your system has important probiotics and prebiotics. Dairy sources include yogurt, kefir, and cottage cheese. Nondairy sources include tofu, soy yogurt, miso, tempe, and sauerkraut.
- Do some exercise—both cardio and strength training. Aim for four times a week, and walk every day.
- Stretching is important. It increases oxygen and blood flow, and decreases stress.

Just remember that there are many wonderful and nutritious foods you can choose from that will help to keep your body cleansed—today, and every day. Using a wide variety of the nutritious foods in your everyday diet is the way to take the best and the most of what the earth has to offer you for your bodily health.

Zucchini Zuper Soup (Gluten-Free)

*This recipe is packed with delicious veggies and flavorful spices,
and is also safe for those who suffer from a gluten allergy.*

INGREDIENTS | YIELDS 1–2 SERVINGS

½ small onion, peeled and chopped

2 stalks celery, chopped

3 cloves garlic, peeled and minced

2–3 teaspoons extra-virgin olive oil

1 mango or ½ cup papaya or pear

2 zucchini, peeled and chopped

½ cup chopped, peeled potato or sweet potato

2 fresh basil leaves

¼ teaspoon nutmeg

Pinch of white pepper or black pepper, or to taste

Pinch of sea salt, or to taste

1¼ cups reduced salt, additive-free vegetable or chicken broth

¼ –½ cup nonfat, plain Greek-style yogurt (optional)

1. In a medium-size saucepan sauté the onion, celery, and garlic in oil to soften for about 3 minutes.

2. Add the fruit, zucchini, potato, basil, seasonings, and broth. Simmer until the vegetables are just tender, about 8 minutes.

3. Cool a little and carefully place in a blender and blend together until smooth. Serve warm or cold.

4. Optional: stir in ¼ cup yogurt after blending.

Pineapple Pear for Reducing Constipation

*Pineapple and pear are naturally sweet fruits that make
this treat easy to love—and easy on your insides!*

INGREDIENTS | YIELDS 1 SERVING

½ cup pineapple

1 pear, cored

1 stalk celery (remove strings)

½ cup chopped kale

1 tablespoon ground flaxseed

1–2 dried, pitted prunes

1 tablespoon wheat germ

1½ cups water, ice as desired

Combine all the ingredients in blender and blend until smooth. Pour into a glass and serve.

Banana Belly Pleaser

This banana treat adds cottage cheese to creamy it up and add lots of protein.

INGREDIENTS | YIELDS 2 SERVINGS

1 banana

½ cup blueberries (optional)

½ cup nonfat, plain yogurt or cottage cheese

½ cup soy or almond milk

1 tablespoon nut butter (almond or peanut)

Cinnamon, to taste

1 cup water, and add ice if desired

Combine all ingredients in a blender and blend until smooth. Pour into a glass and serve.

Fragrant Digestion-Friendly Tofu Asparagus Soup

This soup not only assists in digestion, but smells and tastes yummy!

INGREDIENTS | YIELDS 1 SERVING

1 tablespoon extra-virgin olive oil
1 teaspoon cumin seeds
½ cup chopped asparagus tips
1 cup diced silken tofu
½ teaspoon ground coriander
Sea salt, to taste
½ teaspoon freshly ground black pepper
1 teaspoon chopped fresh cilantro

1. Heat the oil in a nonstick pan and add the cumin seeds.

2. When the seeds turn rich brown and fragrant, in about 1–2 minutes, add the asparagus tips and tofu. Sauté for 4 minutes, gently breaking up the tofu with a spatula.

3. Add the coriander, salt if desired, pepper, and cilantro.

4. Add all to blender and blend until smooth. Serve warm.

Salad in a Glass

Here's a garden full of goodness in a glass.

INGREDIENTS | YIELDS 1 SERVING

1 cup water
4 romaine lettuce leaves
½ tomato
1 small carrot, chopped
½ small beet, chopped
1 stalk celery, chopped
½ cucumber
2 teaspoons extra-virgin olive oil
Juice of ½ lime
1 clove garlic (optional)

1. Put the water into a blender.

2. Add the lettuce leaves and tomato, and blend.

3. Add the remaining ingredients. Blend until smooth. Pour into a glass and serve.

Cream of Squash Soup

This soup was created and recommended for digestion by Gayle Stolove, BS, RN, LMT, macrobiotic educator, personal chef, and founder of Wholly Macro, www.whollymacrobiotics.com.

INGREDIENTS | YIELDS 3–4 SERVINGS

2 cups cubed and peeled squash (butternut, acorn, or kabocha)

1 dried shiitake mushroom, soaked and diced

1 carrot, chopped

1 yellow onion, chopped

1 clove garlic

1 tablespoon unrefined vegetable oil

½ cup water

½ cup soy milk or soy and rice milk blend

1 tablespoon sesame tahini

Soy sauce, to taste (optional)

1. Place squash, carrots, mushrooms, and enough water to just cover into a sauce pan. Cover and boil until soft, about 10 minutes.

2. In separate pan sauté onions, garlic, and oil until carmelized (about 30 minutes).

3. Place squash and onion mixture into blender and blend smooth, adding the ½ cup water and additional water as needed.

4. Place purée in a pot over medium heat. Add the soy milk, and tahini.

5. Whisk until creamy. Add soy sauce to taste.

Be Kind to Your Tummy!

Sweet and orange beta carotene–rich kabocha, butternut, or acorn squash, and naturally sweet yellow onions are known in Eastern medicine to be relaxing to the stomach, spleen, and pancreas. When these organs are soft and relaxed instead of tight and hard, they are better able to perform their respective important functions related to digestion and assimilation, creating a pleasant and stable blood sugar level resulting in a happy state of mind, and sending energy flowing freely throughout the body and mind.

Soothing Barley Mushroom Soup

*This cleanse recipe is perfect for cold evenings or rainy-day lunches,
and is sure to warm you to your toes.*

INGREDIENTS | YIELDS 1–2 SERVINGS

½ onion, chopped
1 stalk celery, chopped
1 carrot, chopped
2 tablespoons barley
2 cups vegetable or chicken broth
½ cup mushrooms
½ cup chopped, peeled potato
or sweet potato
¼ cup chopped watercress
1 cup milk (optional)
Paprika, to taste
Salt and pepper, to taste

1. In a large soup pot, combine the onion, celery, carrot, barley, and broth. Bring to a boil and cook for 30 minutes.

2. Add the mushrooms and potato and cook another 30 minutes.

3. Add the watercress and milk 20 minutes before serving. Season to taste. Blend all ingredients together in a blender and serve warm.

CHAPTER 5

Cleansing for Strength and Stamina

The ability to move is a prize. There are more than 600 muscles in the body, and they do sometimes have limitations on them. But it is an accepted way of life that one should be able to be "up and at 'em"—jump out of bed in the morning, exercise, go through the day, and still have stamina by evening without flopping down, exhausted, powerless, or drained of strength. Dragging around arms that feel like bowling balls or legs that feel like rooted tree trunks—these are not happy experiences.

Typical Muscle Issues

There are times when strength is just gone—for seemingly no reason. But there is a healthy approach you can take that will add to your strength and stamina—whether you want to be an athlete or just want to be able to participate in life's activities better. It is time to find the strength and stamina you need and to tell your brain what to do to make it happen.

FACT

In the old Southwest, American Indian messengers wore bags containing chia seed and bee pollen to eat on long running journeys to sustain a high energy level. According to stories, they sometimes ran close to 250 miles nonstop between Mexico, Tucson, and San Diego. Makes thirty minutes on the treadmill not seem so bad.

Show Your Muscles

Almost all of your muscles work in pairs. That is because muscles can only be used to "pull"; they cannot "push." So when you bend your arm at the elbow, for example, your bicep pulls your arm up, but that same muscle cannot push it back down; that is accomplished by the triceps on the back of your arm pulling it back down in the opposite direction.

Even if you're pushing your shopping cart loaded with groceries with both of your arms, your muscles are actually "pulling" inside of your arms to generate the strength to do so. It is because of this "pulling" action that muscles can become easily strained or "pulled." You see, muscles are made up of fibers, basically strings or strands. You know what happens if you stretch any string long enough: it breaks or tears. The fibers in muscles are subject to similar tearing.

But a pulled muscle isn't the only pain you have to deal with if your muscles aren't up to snuff. You do not have to be a weak, shrinking violet to experience one of the most common issues with muscle function: lack of strength. The medical dictionaries define weakness as just that—"a loss of muscle strength."

Weakness in the Muscles

Much like with strained muscles, the most common cause of weakness in the muscles is overuse of underconditioned muscle. You know the drill: on top of the regular week's activity, on Sunday you decide to take a bike ride, clean the house, and then move a bunch of boxes out of the attic or cellar. You probably felt pretty proud of yourself—until you woke up the next morning and it felt as if the coffee pot weighed a ton. If it feels like someone pulled the plug on the power supply to your arms, you're right—that is pretty much exactly what happened.

When you push out-of-shape muscles to exhaustion, what you are really doing is tearing up the proteins inside the muscle fibers. At full strength and normal functioning, these proteins link together in chains that provide the power that makes muscles flex. And then this lets you lift things, push, pull, and do the countless other movements involved in a day of yard work.

ALERT

Not all protein is the same. Learn to tell the difference between types of protein. High-quality proteins are foods that have all of the building blocks to make muscle tissue and body proteins. These are usually from animal sources and may or may not be lean. Incomplete proteins are plant proteins that may have one or more building block missing, so they should be eaten in combination with other food to form a complete protein source. Plant foods are usually very lean.

But when the proteins get torn from overactivity, they can't link up the right way and form the necessary chains, and then you do not have the power to perform even simple movements. Doctors say that depending on the extent of damage, it can take days for the proteins to be repaired and for your muscles to regain strength.

Obviously, the best way to avoid this is to not overdo it, but it is also important to keep your muscles as toned and fit as possible. Of course, exercise is one way to do that, but the other key to making sure that your muscle strength is there when you need it is to eat the right foods that provide power and build muscle.

Fibromyalgia

Not all muscle pain and weakness is caused by overexertion. If your muscles seem to hurt all the time, regardless of your level of activity, especially in your shoulders, neck and hips, you could be suffering from fibromyalgia. *Fibromyalgia* literally means "pain in the fibrous muscle tissue." So, when a doctor says, "You have *fibromyalgia*, it is really no more of a diagnosis than saying "you have a headache." Many times the causes leading to the types of pain that result in a *fibromyalgia* label can be found right in your daily diet. The pain from fibromyalgia can be debilitating—making it hard for sufferers even to get out of bed and do simple tasks. This inactivity leads to greater muscle breakdown and weakness, and it becomes a vicious cycle.

Chronic Fatigue Syndrome

Related to fibromyalgia is another condition known as chronic fatigue syndrome. Chronic fatigue syndrome, or CFS, is usually given as a diagnosis when someone has suffered unexplainable weakness or tiredness for more than six months. Most doctors agree that it usually starts with a weakened immune system from some kind of viral infection such as the flu. While the exact causes of CFS are vague, it is clear that certain nutritional deficiencies can aggravate the condition. And even if it's not CFS, certainly the toxins in most typical diets do not provide proper nutrition and that leads to muscle weakness and lack of stamina.

You Gotta Have Heart!

A last and important note is that healthy muscle function is not all about how much you can bench press or how sculpted your abs are. Your heart is a muscle too—and a lifestyle that puts strain on your other muscles can do the same to your heart. So, doing things to cleanse and strengthen your other muscles can also have a positive impact on coronary function.

Best Nutrients for Muscles

"Eat your vegetables if you want to grow big and strong." It seems like moms have been saying that to kids for decades. Turns out moms are pretty smart cookies! Vegetables are a primary source of many of the nutrients that are required to build lean, strong muscle. However, veggies aren't the whole story when it comes to increasing strength and reducing muscle pain and fatigue.

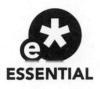

ESSENTIAL

Caffeine in limited amounts and when used properly can be helpful in strengthening muscle and fighting fatigue. Caffeine causes the body to use a larger proportion of fat for fuel instead of stored carbs, so this can increase endurance and stamina.

Proteins are the power behind muscles, and the building blocks of proteins are amino acids. Many of the fundamental muscle-building amino acids are found in various vegetables, but lean meats in many cases are a much more abundant source of these critical strength-enhancing nutrients.

L-carnitine

One important amino acid is L-carnitine. Carnitine is found in just about every cell in your body. The mitochondria of cells are their "energy-producing factories." Fatty acids are the fuel for the power plant. Like your local power company burns coal or natural gas to produce electricity, the mitochondria burns fat to produce energy for life. Carnitine is responsible for bringing the "raw material," the fatty acids, into the mitochondria to be converted into energy. There have been studies that have found that some sufferers of CFS have decreased levels of carnitine. Carnitine deficiency has also been indicated as a reason for muscle fatigue, pain, and impaired exercise tolerance.

Leucine

Another amino acid essential for building strong muscles is leucine. Leucine is one of the key amino acids that are the building blocks of the proteins that make up muscle tissue. Leucine levels are depleted after some types of exercise, and that can be responsible for much of the pain, cramping, and stiffness that follow a workout from aerobics or weights, or sports activities. Increasing dietary intake of leucine can make muscles more tolerant to rigorous exercise. Leucine has also been found to lower blood sugar levels and aids in increasing growth hormone production. Isoleucine and valine are two other amino acids that make up the chain that is the basis for the foundation of muscle protein.

ESSENTIAL

An herbal tea made from horsetail could increase strength and stamina. The herb horsetail contains silica, and increased amounts of silica in the diet have been shown to improve strength and performance.

Lysine

Lysine is another amino acid that is essential for musculoskeletal health and function.

It helps build the long-chain muscle proteins and helps in collagen formation and tissue repair. Lysine has been used to treat people in recovery from sports injuries and surgery.

L-arginine and L-cirtulline

Ask any bodybuilder about strength training, amino acids, and building muscle, and they will surely mention L-arginine and L-citrulline. Arginine and citrulline are amino acids that stimulate the production of nitrous oxide. By increasing nitrous oxide, these amino acids improve blood flow. Better blood flow means greater oxygenation to the muscles, which means that the heart does not have to work as hard. With the heart not needing to pump as strongly for blood flow, you have increased strength and stamina in the other parts of your body. The less of the body's energy that is needed to keep the heart healthy and pumping properly, the more of it that is available for overall strength and stamina.

ATP

Adenosine triphosphate (ATP) is a compound that is an immediate source of energy for the body's cells, especially muscle cells. ATP is made by the body, so it is not a nutrient that you can take in with your diet. But something necessary for it in the body is coenzyme Q10 (CoQ10). Coenzyme Q10 has a most important role in the inner workings of your body and proper muscle function; your body cannot make ATP without CoQ10.

Pump Some Iron

Iron is necessary for the production of red blood cells and therefore has always been linked to building "strong blood," muscle, and combating anemia, a major source of fatigue and weakness.

ESSENTIAL

Magnesium is another mineral that can aid in muscle strength and function. Like potassium, calcium, and sodium, it is an electrolyte. An electrolyte is a substance that helps to transmit electricity. Electrolytes provide power to your car batteries—and in the body, to your muscles!

Take Those Vitamins

There are several vitamins that are necessary for building muscle and fighting fatigue. Vitamin C is important for building collagen; vitamin E helps to reduce muscle soreness, prevent cellular damage, and repair muscle tissue. Vitamin B_{12} has long been shown to reduce tiredness and fatigue. Vitamin C is also a powerful antioxidant that helps to remove free radicals in the blood, which lead to poor oxygenation of cells and increased fatigue and decreased strength.

What to Put in Your Shopping Cart

Here are some foods that are high in the nutrients that can help you with your cleanse. Choose as many of them as you wish, and keep on choosing them even after your cleanse.

- **Protein foods:** eggs, dairy, meat, poultry, fish, beans, nuts, whole grains, and soy products
- **Complex carb foods:** whole grains, legumes, fruits, and vegetables
- **Healthy fat foods:** omega-3 and omega-6—tuna, salmon, seeds, nuts, flaxseed, walnuts, sardines, halibut, snapper, shrimp, and scallops
- **Amino acid–rich foods:** cottage cheese, fish, seafood, meat, poultry, nuts, peanuts, brown rice, lentils, sesame seeds, avocado, tempeh, and wheat germ
- **Blood-building foods:** spinach, wheat grass, raisins, prunes, kidney beans, mushrooms, apricots, soy foods, ginger, citrus fruits, and alfalfa
- **Vitamin and mineral rich foods:** eggs, sardines, beef, lamb, wheat germ, spinach, broccoli, cauliflower, Brussels sprouts, turnips, celery, carrots, cabbage, asparagus, kale, lettuce, cucumbers, tomatoes, garlic, onions, peanuts, mushrooms, leafy greens, artichokes, lima beans, lentils, potatoes, raisins, prunes, apples, bananas, all berries, all melons, grapes, plums, cranberries, brewer's yeast, rice, wheat bran, wheat germ, tofu, and tempeh
- **Vitamin A foods:** citrus fruit, tomatoes, carrots, mango, red bell peppers, spinach, collard greens, sweet potatoes, kale, turnip greens, Swiss chard, milk, and eggs
- **Vitamin B foods:** spinach, bell peppers, turnip greens, garlic, cauliflower, celery, cabbage, asparagus, mushrooms, broccoli, collard greens, Brussels sprouts, turmeric, tuna, cod, salmon, snapper, halibut, chicken, calf liver, and turkey breast
- **Vitamin C foods:** citrus fruits, strawberry, lemon, papaya, grapefruit, cantaloupe, raspberry, watermelon, pineapple, parsley, broccoli, red and green bell peppers, cauliflower, mustard greens, kiwi, snow peas, and zucchini
- **Magnesium and folate foods:** beans, turmeric, spinach, squash, mustard greens, pumpkin, soybeans, sunflower seeds, flaxseeds, sesame

seeds, green beans, cucumbers, celery, kale, black and navy beans, peppermint, and molasses

- **Iron foods:** soybeans, lentils, spinach, tofu, sesame seeds, kidney beans, pumpkin seeds, garbanzo and navy beans, chard, romaine, thyme, turmeric, string beans, shiitake mushrooms, and molasses
- **CoQ10 foods:** organ meats, including liver, heart, and kidney, fish, whole grains, and wheat germ

FACT

The egg is a very high-quality source of protein, and the protein source that is most similar to our body's own. One regular size egg contains only 5 grams of fat, a mere 70 calories, and 280 mg of cholesterol. It can be easily fit into a healthy diet even if you are watching your waistline.

How a Cleanse Can Help

You need your muscles to give you movement, and the extra push you need for endurance is all affected by what you eat. Certain foods and ways of eating can actually reduce your stamina and strength, and no doubt some or many of those have been in your system. A cleanse for strength and stamina will help to give your body a rest and a change from some of the de-energizing problems of valueless non-nutrient foods that have been in your body. It will be a start-off point to begin giving your body and muscles the particular attention they need. Just think of your body as your beautiful transport machine: a car or space vehicle—use your imagination. If your vehicle doesn't have a golden tank of fuel, it will peter out.

The day before your cleanse, plan your next day with two small activities you would be pleased to do—whether it be walking to the mailbox or doing an exercise video, or a two-minute yoga stretch, or a few lifts of hand weights while looking out the window.

Begin your day with a large glass of water with a squirt of lime or lemon; drink slowly, taking the time for some deep, easy breathing. If you feel the energy for five minutes of stretches, do so; otherwise, first take in some nutrients, such as 1 tablespoon of wheat germ or oat bran mixed in ⅓ cup soy or skim milk or yogurt with 1 teaspoon of raisins.

FACT

> Vitamin C in clinical trials has been shown to reduce muscle soreness after exercise. Researchers at one chiropractic college gave 3,000mg of vitamin C to one group of students and placebos to another. Evaluating both groups after three days, it was found that the students in the vitamin C group developed significantly less muscle soreness after exercising than the group that took the placebos.

Choose three nutrient-rich meals for breakfast, lunch, and dinner, and two small nutrient snacks in between. In-between snacks can include combinations of complex carbs and protein such as wheat germ with soy milk or yogurt and a small amount of raisins or pear or pineapple. If you have problems relaxing and sleeping, you may wish to include an after-dinner snack, such as 1–2 stalks of celery puréed in a blender with ½ cup water, ½ carrot (optional), and 1 teaspoon of honey (optional). Make sure to include at least eight glasses of water or herb teas throughout the day. Plan to do your cleanse for one to three days. Some suggested recipes can be found at the end of th chapter.

After the Cleanse

Following your cleanse, here are some things to keep in mind:

- Keep your drinking/flushing habits alive with herbal teas and water.
- Always make sure your system has important probiotics and prebiotics. Dairy sources include yogurt, kefir, and cottage cheese. Nondairy sources include tofu, soy yogurt, miso, tempe, and sauerkraut.
- Remember that there are many wonderful and nutritious foods you can choose from that will help keep your body cleansed—today, and every day. Using a wide variety of foods in your everyday diet is the way to take the best and the most of what the earth has to offer.

- Do some exercise—both cardio and strength training. Aim for four times a week, and walk every day.
- Stretching is important. It increases oxygen and blood flow, and decreases stress.

When you get back to your everyday routine, here are some points to keep in mind: Eat and enjoy a wide variety of healthy foods to make sure your body gets the important nutrients for your muscles that are found in not just a limited few foods. Always start off your day with a healthy breakfast to get the energy and muscles going and the stamina you need throughout the day. Protein is the building block for all tissues, particularly muscle. Whole grains contain amino acids, the building blocks of protein that really help build muscle and increase your stamina.

FACT

Looking for healthy, nutritious, and high-protein snacks? Some easy ways to get low-glycemic, lean protein on-the-go are fat-free yogurt, especially Greek style, mozzarella cheese, hard-boiled eggs, or edamame.

Avoid simple carbohydrates like sugars and white flour that just spike your blood sugar. Keep your fats the healthy ones. It's been discovered that membranes that have polyunsaturated fats in them are vulnerable to free radical attack. Eating the right way will mean that muscle and red blood cells will be more resistant to damage.

Avoid processed food and foods with additives. Use whole foods as much as possible. For example, processed orange juice often has added sugars; instead, choose a whole orange. Try to choose organic fruits and vegetables. Many other fruits and vegetables are highly contaminated with pesticides. Fiber is important to get the digestive bowels moving daily, as constipation can bring on low energy. Sprinkling flaxseeds on foods is a great way to add fiber.

Train with weights—even light training is one way to stimulate the growth of muscle tissue. When you do exercise, choose a mini-snack about thirty to sixty minutes before exercising to give you the energy to "go." If you do not have enough nutrition to exercise, it can cause dizziness and fatigue—and you don't want that when you are trying to build strength and stamina. The kinds of choices for a mini-meal could include low-fat yogurt or cottage cheese and a banana, string cheese and an apple, or peanut or nut butter on a cracker.

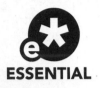

ESSENTIAL

After any intense workout, "sports drinks" can be a choice other than water to rehydrate. Too much water can actually further deplete already lost electrolytes. Many sports drinks have been designed to replace electrolytes and have added potassium and sodium.

After exercise, drink a glass of water. It can be dangerous to drink extra-large quantities of water at one time because it can dilute your electrolyte levels and cause physical problems, but do remember to keep sipping throughout your workout and afterward, even if you aren't thirsty.

Get enough rest and sleep. The body and the muscles need their time to rest and repair and grow strong. Lack of proper sleep or not enough sleep at all make up the majority of sleep problems that most people face. Too much sleep is another problem! Sleep until you feel rested, and make sure you keep your body on that sleep schedule—even on the weekends.

Spinach So Strong Soup

*Spinach has long been an enemy of vegetable-haters everywhere,
but this recipe makes it appealing to even the most anti-spinach cleanser!*

INGREDIENTS | YIELDS 1 SERVING

1 cup spinach
2 stalks celery (remove strings)
1 tomato
¼ cup mushrooms
½ cup tofu
1 teaspoon fresh basil
¼ cup chopped fresh parsley
¼ cup chopped onion
½ clove garlic
1 teaspoon ground flaxseed
1 teaspoon nutritional yeast
¼ cup pine nuts
½ cup soy milk
1 cup water
Sea salt and ground black pepper,
to taste

1. Combine all ingredients in a blender and blend until smooth. Pour into a glass and serve.

2. May be served warm, so if you prefer that, transfer mixture to a pot over the stove and heat until a drop feels warm on the back of your hand.

Cauliflower Can Do Soup

This scrumptious soup is packed with the power of cauliflower,
and can give you the stamina to take on the day.

INGREDIENTS | YIELDS 1–2 SERVINGS

1 cup cauliflower florets

1 carrot

1 cup chopped romaine

¼ cup chopped parsley

¼ cup chopped onion

¼ cup mushrooms

1 teaspoon ground flaxseed

1 tablespoon nutritional brewer's yeast

¼ cup cashews or pine nuts

½ cup soy milk

1 cup water

Sea salt and ground black pepper, to taste

1. Place all the ingredients in a blender and blend until smooth. Pour into a glass and serve.

2. May be served warm. Transfer from the blender to a pot on the stove and simmer until a drop feels warm to the back of your hand.

Broccoli Boost Soup

Broccoli is a veggie that is good for energy and tastes great.

INGREDIENTS | YIELDS 1 SERVING

1 cup broccoli florets

½ cup frozen lima beans, cooked slightly to soften

½ cup green beans

2 sprigs parsley

¼ cup chopped onion

½ clove garlic

¼ cup sunflower seeds

1 tablespoon nutritional brewer's yeast

1 teaspoon ground flaxseed

½ cup water

Sea salt and ground black pepper, to taste

1. Combine all the ingredients in a blender and blend until smooth. Pour into a glass and serve.

2. May be served warm. Transfer from the blender to a pot on the stove and simmer until a drop feels warm on the back of your hand.

Fruit and Nut Power Beverage

Fruits and nuts are an excellent but overlooked source of protein.
People often forget that they contain this beneficial nutrient.

INGREDIENTS | YIELDS 1 SERVING

½ cup liquid egg whites

2 tablespoons unsweetened protein powder (whey or soy)

2 teaspoons ground flaxseeds

½ cup strawberries or blueberries

½ banana

1 teaspoon almond butter

1 tablespoon wheat germ

1–2 dried prunes or dates

1 cup water

3–5 ice cubes, depending on desired "iciness"

Combine all the ingredients in a blender and blend until smooth. Pour into a glass and serve.

Almondy Apple Beverage

Two healthy "A"s for you.

INGREDIENTS | YIELDS 1 SERVING

1 cup soy milk

1 (2-ounce) scoop protein powder

¼ cup almonds (soaked in water to soften)

1–2 dried prunes or dates

1 apple, cored

1 teaspoon ground flaxseed

1 tablespoon wheat germ

Cinnamon, to taste (optional)

1 cup water

3–5 ice cubes, depending on iciness desired

Combine all the ingredients in a blender and blend until smooth. Pour into a glass and serve.

CHAPTER 6

Cleansing for Peak Performance at Any Age

Whether you're sitting passively reading in a spare moment in the doctor's office, in your car in traffic checking your GPS or BlackBerry, or taking a chance at a new class on guitar—you want energy. A dull brain, a sluggish body, a weak will, a cold in the nose, or pain in the knee holds you back no matter what you're doing. And to be sure, this is the age of moving forward—fast. But all of these fast conveniences have actually slowed you down by making you use your muscles less.

Typical Energy Issues

Superheroes are part of growing up, and the inspiration they give just doesn't leave you. At one time or another just about everyone pretended to be a Wonder Woman or Green Lantern, with that same tireless, unlimited energy to do great feats. Well, it may not be possible for you to be a superhero, but it would be great to always feel strong and healthy and up to the challenge of today's evil "energy thieves," including the flu, cancers, diabetes, and poor nutrition. And it would be terrific to not have to worry about canceling out on something you really want to do because of "not feeling up to it."

FACT

Physicians and scientists that study aging now agree that 75 percent of an individual's health after age forty is more dependent upon what the person has done to his or her genes, not the genes themselves. In other words, environmental factors such as diet and lifestyle are what makes for peak health.

The research and evidence of what you can do and not do, to keep yourself energized, to be at your peak performance at any age, is proving that it is in your hands. And it doesn't take a magic lasso or a power ring, just a trip to the grocery store and a change of your buying and eating habits.

You Are What You Eat—Really!

Tick, tick, tick. . . . No matter what you do the clock ticks by, you grow older, and the years take their inevitable toll. You may never be able to stop that clock, but you can take measures to slow it down a bit and be your best at any age. Did you know that recent research indicates that Mother Nature has actually programmed human beings to live to be about 120 years old? But most people never get anywhere near that age—and the primary reason? The way they eat.

Degenerative diseases, what you most often think of as the signs of aging—weakness, fatigue, lack of energy, decreased vitality, joint pain, back pain, and even the greater tendency to serious illness such as stroke, heart disease, etc.—are all a part of cellular damage. That's because you are made up of billions and billions of cells that interact in that complicated dance of life. Your greatest enemy that wants to slow down that dance is oxidative stress caused by free radicals. You have no doubt heard about the benefits of antioxidants, That name actually means the cessation of oxidation. Just like the oxidative process that causes metal to rust and eventually break down, free radicals do the same to the cells of the body.

Free Radicals

Free radicals are molecules that tear apart and ravage the cells and tissue of the body just like rust does to your car. Research has suggested that an average cell is subjected to as many as 20 billion "attacks" by free radicals every day.

Normal aging is the regular and expected wear and tear based on your programmed timetable. Typical breakdown issues, stiffness, pain, weakness, lack of energy, are really faster aging and premature breakdown due to improper maintenance. Think of it this way: You would never expect your car to run smoothly at over 100,000 miles if you never changed the oil. So, fixing your diet and lifestyle to lessen any damage done by free-radical buildup is like a good oil change.

Many people think that a general loss of energy and aches and pains in the joints and other parts of the body will just become part of daily life as they get older. But nothing could be further from the truth. Did you ever go to a classic car show? See how sleek and powerful and well preserved some of those "antique" cars are? It's all because their owners have treated them over the years with the utmost care and love. That's what kind of treatment your body needs, too.

ALERT

You don't have to be "old" to experience the problems of aging based on a poor diet. Studies have shown an alarming increase in the levels of cholesterol in teens and children. You are never too young to put down the pizza and pick up the broccoli!

To create good health, rejuvenation, and greater vitality on a cellular level, you have to eat and live to do two things: avoid or lessen cell damage, and feed yourself what will help cellular growth and repair. Greater cellular vitality means more energy is made for all of the body's metabolic processes. In Chinese medicine, they would call this "chi," "life force," or "vital energy"—but no matter what you call it, it is possible to slow the decline of vitality through proper diet and lifestyle.

Best Nutrients for Creating Productive Energy

So what is the best fuel to put in that tank to keep it going strong and running smoothly mile after mile? Peak-performance nutrients break down into a few different categories. But, the main one is the family of antioxidants. Antioxidants are as many as the colors of the rainbow, and in fact that is a good way to look at them, because looking for Mother Nature's bright brilliant colors is a great way to find some of the best antioxidants for vitality and better health and performance. These are the phytonutrients that are responsible for giving fruits and vegetables their different colors. They are also powerful age-defying antioxidants.

ESSENTIAL

Living a long and healthy life requires a balanced diet, but not necessarily the balance you are familiar with. Nutritionists suggest that a balanced "antiaging" diet consist of a 50/25/25 ratio of carbohydrate, protein, fat. As always, processed "white carbs" should be avoided and the carbohydrate components should come from fruits and vegetables. It is suggested that proteins should also be primarily from plant sources such as beans and tofu, with a maximum of one-third from animal sources.

Go Green

Getting your green vegetables is good for you for a number of reasons. One of the first things you notice is what gives them their green color: chlorophyll.

On the molecular level chlorophyll is almost the same as hemoglobin. Hemoglobin is what is responsible for building red blood cells and moving oxygen out of the blood. Chlorophyll not only has a powerful antioxidative effect (cleansing the blood of extra oxygen and free radicals), but it also helps to build red blood cells and fight anemia—a common cause of loss of vitality. Deep-green veggies also contain folate and folic acid, which are both blood-building antioxidants.

FACT

Green leafy vegetables like spinach, kale, and Swiss chard are not only great sources of antioxidants, but they also contain high levels of vitamin K, which helps keep bones strong, and lutein and zeaxanthin, which together can combat vision problems that come with aging.

Orange You Glad?

The carotenoids that give yellow and orange superfoods like squash, pumpkins, and, of course, carrots their color are also powerful antioxidants. Carotenoids aid in the sweeping-out process of cholesterol and protect the linings of cells from oxidative damage.

Also in this yellow band of the "antioxidant rainbow" is curcuma. It is the phytonutrient that makes curry and turmeric yellow. Turmeric is considered a super-antioxidant. It is one of the fundamental curative compounds in Ayurvedic (traditional Indian medicine). Turmeric has been proven in many modern clinical trials to have a powerful anti-inflammatory effect and has been used to treat arthritis.

Red and Purple

Looking at the red/purple part of the spectrum there is the xanthophylls and anthocyanins. Xanthophylls are found in all types of red and yellow peppers and chilies. They are powerful antioxidants, and they have been shown to improve the strength of cell walls. Anthocyanins are responsible for the red, purple, and bluish colors in food and are what gives blueberries, raspberries, and blackberries their powerful antioxidative abilities.

Other colorful phytonutrients are a group called *flavonoids*, which have all been linked to antiaging and overall health. These include isoflavone, quercetin, gingerol, and perhaps the most important of the group, resveratrol. Resveratrol is what gives red wine its color, and it is believed to be the reason for the antioxidant and fat-busting power of red wine that explains the low level of heart disease among the French, even though they eat a high-fat diet.

ESSENTIAL

Sure, fruits and veggies are chock-full of antioxidants—but they are not the only source. Recent research has found that the polyphenols found in whole-grain cereals also lower oxidative stress and offer other antiaging benefits as well. Grape juice is another great source of polyphenols.

Your Own Nutrient Army

If trying to stay youthful and keeping up peak energy at every age can be thought of as a war on free radicals, then the various types of nutrients can be thought of as different divisions of the opposing army. Just like it takes the Army, Air Force, and Navy, each with their own special skills to win a war, no one group of antioxidants can "do it all." Another group of antioxidants proven to fight free radicals are essential vitamins and minerals, especially vitamins A, C, and E, and supporting minerals such as copper, selenium, magnesium, and zinc.

FACT

In ancient Rome, gladiators were known as *hordearii*, which means "eaters of barley." Barley played an important role in ancient Greek culture as well, with the first Olympians attributing much of their strength and athletic prowess to their barley-containing training diets.

The next group in the army of antioxidants and age-fighting nutrients are the amino acids. One leading the charge is acetyl-L-carnitine. Acetyl-L-carnitine not only is a major amino acid that helps move fatty acids out of the blood and into the cells for greater energy and stamina, but it is also antioxidative and protects cells. If L-carnitine is the general, then alpha lipoic acid is second in command. Alpha lipoic acid has long been called the "universal antioxidant." It also helps to replenish other antioxidants such as vitamin E. Two others in this group are phenolic acid, and phytic acid, both found in cereals and whole grains. Phenylalanine is another amino acid that has been found to have several antiaging effects, including lessening of arthritis-related pain.

FACT

A study published in the *Journal of the American Medical Association* found that women who ate diets high in grains, vegetables, fruits, and lean meats were 30 percent less likely to die of any cause than women who didn't eat these foods.

And finally there are the "Special Forces" such as CoQ10. Though neither a phytonutrient, amino acid, or even a vitamin or mineral, CoQ10 is a vital nutrient in the war on aging and free radicals.

What to Put in Your Shopping Cart

Here are some of the foods with the excellent nutrients that can help you with your cleanse, and always for your healthful living. Choose as many as you wish now, and keep on choosing them!

- **Cruciferous vegetables:** broccoli, cauliflower, carrots, turnip, watercress, Brussels sprouts, kale, cabbage, and radishes
- **Anti-inflammatory foods:** nuts, seeds, acai fruit, green foods, sprouts, yogurt, barley, garlic, onion, shallots, chives, beans, lentils, and buckwheat
- **Healthy fats:** olive and canola oil, olives, nuts, seeds, fish, seafood, peanut butter, and avocados
- **Flavonoid-rich foods:** green tea, apples, cranberries, ginger, blueberries, blackberries, raspberries, strawberries, citrus fruits, cabbage, eggplant, buckwheat, parsley, and tomatoes
- **Proteins:** lean meat, poultry, fish, eggs, dairy, and soy products

- **Enzyme-rich foods:** red meat, sardines, codfish, eggs, lamb, spinach, broccoli, peanuts, wheat germ, tempeh, whey, milk products, avocado, and whole grains
- **Foods with vitamin B:** spinach, bell peppers, turnip greens, garlic, cauliflower, celery, cabbage, asparagus, mushrooms, broccoli, collard greens, Brussels sprouts, turmeric, tuna, cod, salmon, snapper, halibut, chicken, calf liver, and turkey breast
- **Foods with vitamin C:** citrus fruits, strawberry, lemon, papaya, grapefruit, cantaloupe, raspberry, watermelon, pineapple, barley, broccoli, red and green bell peppers, cauliflower, mustard greens, kiwi, snow peas, and zucchini
- **Foods with vitamin E:** mustard greens, Swiss chard, spinach, olives, turnip greens, sunflower seeds, almonds, papaya, and blueberries
- **Foods with CoQ10:** fish, liver, heart, kidney, wheat germ, and whole grains
- **Foods with lipoic acid:** broccoli, spinach, collard greens, Swiss chard, calf liver, round steak, and brewer's yeast
- **Foods with carnitine:** beef, milk, codfish, chicken, and Cheddar cheese
- **Foods with potassium:** cabbage, tomatoes, cantaloupe, lima beans, avocados, cucumbers, celery, kale, soybeans, and seeds including sesame, sunflower, and pumpkin
- **Foods with magnesium:** Swiss chard, spinach, yellow squash, broccoli, mustard greens, and basil
- **Foods with resveratrol:** red grapes, wine, grape juice, peanuts, blueberries, and bilberries

ESSENTIAL

"Keep it real" if you want to get the most antiaging and invigorating benefits from your food. The more a food is processed, the lower it's content of fiber, vitamins, minerals, and phytonutrients—and the higher the percentage of fat and calories!

How a Cleanse Can Help

So, you want to find and maintain your peak performance now and in the years to come. With renewed strength also comes renewed vitality and a "can do" attitude to seize the day! You want your days uninterrupted by health setbacks. A cleanse for peak performance can change a path that could be blocked, a dead end, and open up a new, easy path. A cleanse for peak performance will help make your mountains as reachable as molehills and put your personal, professional, and physical peaks right within easy reach!

ESSENTIAL

Research has found that vitamin D plays a key role in muscle strength and that vitamin D deficiency has been linked to muscle weakness and fatigue. It is believed that a lack of vitamin D leads to a buildup of fat in the muscles that inhibits performance. Other than milk that has been fortified with vitamin D, excellent sources of vitamin D include salmon, sardines, and shrimp.

Begin your day with a large glass of water with a squirt of lemon or lime juice. Choose a breakfast, lunch, and dinner from the recipes below. You may choose two snacks in between meals. You can also sip on a glass of water with a blend of 1 or 2 ounces of watermelon, cantaloupe, or cucumber, and add ¼ cup yogurt and/or ¼ cup soaked nuts or seeds if you like. Be sure to drink eight to ten glasses of fluids a day using herbal teas and water. Aim to do your cleanse for one to three days.

After the Cleanse

Following your cleanse, here are some things to keep in mind:

- Begin to increase your selection and amounts of solid foods and amounts. A great interim meal is chickpeas or garbanzo beans, cooked and simmered in a sauce of tomatoes, curry spices, and chopped walnuts, with brown rice.

- Always make sure your system has important probiotics and prebiotics. Dairy sources include yogurt, kefir, and cottage cheese. Nondairy sources include tofu, soy yogurt, miso, tempeh, and sauerkraut.
- Keep your drinking/flushing habits alive with herbal teas and water.
- Do some exercise—both cardio and strength training. Aim for four times a week, and walk every day.
- Stretching is important. It increases oxygen and blood flow, and decreases stress.

ALERT

Women are at much greater risk of osteoporosis than men are, so they need more calcium. But all that dairy may not be so good for the waistline. Try veggie sources of calcium instead, such as beans, broccoli, kale, Brussels sprouts, and collard greens. Not only do they build bones, but they have some powerful antioxidants too.

Remember that there are many, many wonderful and nutritious foods you can choose from that will help to keep your body at peak performance—today, and in the future. Using a wide variety of foods in your everyday diet is the way to take the best and the most of what the earth has to offer.

By making the right food choices you have learned how to add years to your life—and life to your years!

A Soup That Beets All

Beets are given a bad rap in the veggie community,
but the nutrients they provide can keep you performing at a high level.

INGREDIENTS | YIELDS 1–2 SERVINGS

1½ cups water

¼ cup basmati rice, washed and rinsed several times

½ cup peeled and grated beets

½ cup grated carrot

1 cup greens (kale, spinach)

½ teaspoon minced gingerroot

⅛ teaspoon ground cumin

⅛ teaspoon ground coriander

½ clove garlic minced (optional)

¼ cup ground walnuts

Sea salt and ground black pepper, to taste (optional)

1. Bring the water to a boil in a medium sized pot. Add the rice, vegetables, walnuts, and spices.

2. Turn heat to low, cover, and simmer 60–80 minutes.

3. Add salt and pepper to taste, if desired. Cool a little first, then carefully place the mixture in a blender and blend until smooth. Serve warm.

Turnip Sipping Soup

Often partnered with the carrot, turnips have long been a staple of Thanksgiving and other holidays, but this root veggie is delicious anytime!

INGREDIENTS | YIELDS 2 SERVINGS

¾ cup peeled, diced carrot

½ cup peeled, diced turnips

½ cup diced celery

2 tablespoons barley, washed and soaked

¼ teaspoon ground cumin

½ clove garlic (optional)

2 teaspoons extra-virgin olive oil

2 cups vegetable broth

1 tablespoon chopped fresh parsley

1. In a large frying pan over medium heat sauté the vegetables, soaked barley, cumin, and garlic in olive oil 3–4 minutes.

2. Add the broth and simmer 20 minutes, or until tender.

3. Cool a little then carefully place the mixture with the parsley in a blender and blend smooth. Serve immediately.

Green and Nutty Beverage

Here's a beverage that gives you your greens, and some protein to carry you along.

INGREDIENTS | YIELDS 1 SERVING

1 cup kale or spinach (or a mix), trimmed and washed

1 carrot

¼ cup soaked almonds

1 teaspoon chopped fresh basil

1 tablespoon ground flaxseeds

1 cup water

Ice cubes to desired level of "iciness" (optional)

Combine all the ingredients in a blender and blend until smooth. Pour into a glass and serve.

Cottage Cheese Pink or Blue Beverage

This recipe can play to your tastes: if you are a blueberry fan,
you can use those for a blue treat, or if you prefer the strawberry, those can be substituted.

INGREDIENTS | YIELDS 1 SERVING

1 cup water
2 tablespoons wheat germ
⅓ cup fat free or low fat cottage cheese
½ banana
1 pitted red date or 1 pitted prune
⅔ cup strawberries or blueberries

1. In a small bowl, combine the water and wheat germ. Let sit for 15 minutes.

2. Add all the ingredients, including the wheat germ and the water it is in, to a blender. Blend until smooth. Pour into a glass and serve.

Berries for Long Life Beverage

*This "berry" good recipe offers the alternative of strawberries,
blueberries, or an assortment of berries. If you have trouble choosing, use them all!*

INGREDIENTS | YIELDS 1 SERVING

1 cup water

2 tablespoons wheat germ

1 cup blueberries, strawberries, or mixed berries

1 red date, pitted, or 1 pitted prune

1 (2-ounce) scoop whey or soy protein powder

1 cup almond, rice, or soy milk, or 1 cup plain, nonfat or lowfat yogurt

1 teaspoon ground flaxseed

2–3 ice cubes, or to taste for desired "iciness"

1. In a small bowl, combine the water and wheat germ, and let sit for 10 minutes.

2. Add all ingredients to the blender, including the wheat germ and water, and blend until smooth. Pour into a glass and serve.

Fruit and Minty Green Beverage

The flavor of mint is a great palate cleanser, and it makes you feel fresh and clean.

INGREDIENTS | YIELDS 1 SERVING

1 pear

½ banana

½ orange

1 cup chopped kale

2 tablespoons chopped fresh mint

1 teaspoon ground flaxseed

¼ cup ground cashews

2–3 ice cubes or as desired for level of "iciness"

1½ cups water

1 dried, pitted prune

Place all the ingredients in a blender and blend until smooth. Pour into a glass and serve.

Don't Lose Your Tempeh

Adding 2 ounces of tempeh to your blended soups or drinks adds great nutrients for peak energy, including protein and important carnitine enzymes. Some tempeh comes ready to eat, while others must be cooked first. Make sure the tempeh is very fresh, with no "off" flavor. If you are not sure about the quality of tempeh you should first steam it for 10 minutes and let it cool. Mixing it with a little water first will help with the smoothness.

CHAPTER 7

Cleansing for Clearer Skin and Stronger Nails

People who look beautiful have a glow—whether they do or don't have ideal features, that certain glow radiates beauty. Much of that glow comes from clear, healthy skin, nails, and hair. When you see a person, the first thing you usually notice is his or her face. And then when you meet a person, shake hands, and talk, you often notice his or her nails.

Typical Skin Disorders and Issues

Most people have been in the situation where they're talking to a person, but instead of paying attention to what's being said, the person's pimples, sores, spots, blemishes, veins, and discoloration become unfortunate points of focus. Or, the situation where a fun activity is deadened for a moment by the exclamation "geesh, I just broke my nail." For sure, stronger nails and clearer skin make for a beautiful experience all the way around.

What do people do to try to get clearer skin and stronger nails? Often, people try to mask the problems with creams and makeup and various coverings. But such products can often make problems worse, and at best, they are only a temporary solution. Your skin—which includes your nails and hair—is the largest organ of your body. So what you really need is not just a temporary covering, but something that will repair your skin as a whole. The main issue regarding skin care is how to keep skin looking healthy and youthful at any age.

Skin and the Aging Process

There are many reasons why the skin ages; probably the number one outside factor is sun exposure. Physical stress, environmental issues such as pollution, and smoking can all cause skin to age. And, as you age there's a gravitational pull on your skin that, unfortunately, just cannot be helped.

ALERT

For truly healthy skin you must minimize your exposure to UVA and UVB radiation, not only to prevent skin cancer, but also to reduce the appearance of aging skin. Always wear sunscreen with at least an SPF of 15 and try to avoid being in the sun when UV is at its peak—between the hours of 10 A.M. and 4 P.M.

While the skin is under attack from all of these external forces, it is also true that when it comes to healthy skin, what is going on inside is just as important as the outside. In other words, good skin care and protection from all of those ravages of the elements begins under the surface of the skin—inside your body. As people age the skin's ability to fix damage and renew itself lessens. And, there is a natural loss of the elements in the skin. As years go by, the skin becomes less elastic and supple; it becomes thinner and dryer. It can be injured easier and heals more slowly.

Skin is not only the body's largest organ; it is also a very important one, and not just to the way you look. Your skin is nature's precious gift that is there as a shield from dangerous pathogens that would and could enter the body, such as viruses and bacteria. Skin helps to keep you cool and regulates body temperature, and it has the purpose of protecting you from its worst enemy—the sun's rays.

ESSENTIAL

Ever see a carrot with sunburn? No? Well, you probably never will. Nutrients in carrots give them a natural sunscreen, and if you have light skin, eating them provides the same to you, with a sunscreen protection equal to 2–4 SPF.

Skin care professionals agree that there really is not a Fountain of Youth, but you are never too old or too young to start on good skin care. There are many ways to keep your skin looking as beautiful as possible—at any age. We've all heard the expression "you are what you eat." It certainly applies to having and keeping youthful and healthy skin. A skin healthy diet can do a lot to replace what normal aging and nature itself takes out.

The Basics of Skin

The skin is basically divided into three layers: the epidermis, the dermal layer, and the hypodermis. The epidermis is the outermost layer of the skin. It is the actual barrier between the body and the outside world. The next layer down is the dermis. It is the layer of the skin where the smaller blood vessels that feed the epidermis are found. The dermis is where elastin and collagen are found, which gives the skin its firmness and structure. The deepest layer of the skin, the hypodermis, sometimes called the *subcutaneous layer*, is where the main sweat glands, hair follicles, and major blood vessels that feed your skin are found.

When the renewing process of the epidermis slows, there is not as good an exchange of nutrients and vital energies between the layers. Removal of waste, including free radicals, slows down. The lowered amounts of nutrients leads to less collagen being made, and an ongoing cycle of deterioration ensues.

As super-oxide radicals build up, these molecules eat away at healthy collagen like an acid. Collagen is the primary fiber that supports the skin. When there is a certain amount of collagen gone, the result is lines, wrinkles, and sagging. The breakdown and aging of skin is mostly caused by oxidation. And the easiest way to prevent or lessen oxidation in the body is to eat a diet rich in antioxidants.

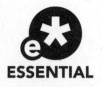

ESSENTIAL

The anthocyanins in pomegranates have been shown to strengthen vein walls. One of the many antiaging benefits of drinking pomegranate juice is the reduction of the appearance of spider veins.

In addition to a general loss of elasticity and those dreaded "lines and wrinkles," two other major worries about skin are age spots and varicose veins. Age spots are those brownish patches that pop up on almost everyone's skin over time. They are caused by sun exposure. Actually, "age spots" is a misleading name, because they really have nothing to do with how old you are, but rather with how much or how long you are in the sun. As you get older, the time you have been in the sun has also been longer, so they tend to appear later in life. "Sun spots" would be a better name.

Veins

Varicose veins and spider veins, a smaller form of the same condition, are veins that have become twisted due to engorged blood, and swollen blood vessels. Usually appearing on the legs, varicose veins can be unattractive. There are also situations where they can be painful and debilitating. The appearance of both age spots and varicose veins can also be lessened with a skin healthy diet.

Acne and Psoriasis

Acne is a common skin condition due to the overproduction of oil by the oil glands of the skin that is normally used to lubricate the skin. Extra oil gets trapped and blocks up oil ducts and results in pimples, blackheads, and whiteheads on the surface of skin. It may be popular belief that acne affects only teens, but this is not the case—it can be a skin problem for anyone, at any age.

ALERT

Concentrating on just one skin-friendly nutrient, such as vitamin A, is never a good idea. Proper skin care needs balance—a good mix of the nutrients known to contribute to overall skin health. Each nutrient provides distinct types of defenses for healthy skin. For example, tissue generation, mucous membrane strength, and collagen synthesis are helped by vitamins A and C. Free-radical damage is best dealt with by a good supply of vitamin E and plant flavonoids. For clearer and great skin, eat a variety of skin healthy foods.

Psoriasis is a chronic skin disease that is very common. Psoriasis is seen as patches of raised red skin with thick, silvery scales, which can be itchy and sometimes painful.

The good news is that many of the dietary steps you can take to keep skin healthy, moist, and youthful can also help with these conditions. In fact, there are specific diets that can minimize the symptoms of both acne and psoriasis.

Best Nutrients for Your Skin and Nails

The two most important dietary things you can do to keep your skin healthy is good hydration, and to lessen as much as possible the oxidative decay caused by free radicals.

Hydration starts with drinking a lot of water of course, but water isn't the only thing that helps to keep skin moist below the surface. Another key to hydration and youthful looking skin is eating foods rich in the "good fats."

Omega-3s, along with other fatty acids and monounsaturated fats, are good for your body for many reasons. One important benefit is these fats help build a layer of healthy fat below the surface of the skin that locks in moisture. Not all fat is bad fat!

The three most important antioxidants for skin care are vitamins A, C, and E. A study recently published in the *Journal of Investigative Dermatology* reported that increased levels of vitamins C and E in the long term lessen the severity of sunburns from exposure to UVB radiation. Further, the study concluded that the antioxidant vitamins help protect against cellular damage that leads to skin aging. Vitamin A has also been shown to be helpful in lessening the appearance of age spots.

"B" Good

In addition to vitamins A, C, and E, vitamin B complex is also most important for healthy skin. There are several "B" vitamins, and for skin health the most important one is biotin. Biotin is a nutrient essential to the makeup of hair, skin, and nails. Biotin deficiency leads to several skin and nail problems, such as dermatitis and weak, discolored nails.

ALERT

If you are not getting enough zinc, your skin may let you know! Zinc prevents dry, itchy skin and can lessen outbreaks of skin conditions such as eczema, psoriasis, and "winter skin." So, when it comes to holiday meals, skip any greasy dressings and sauces, and have a little extra helping of turkey; it's a food that contains zinc—as do oysters and other lean meats.

In fact, a study found that 2.5mg of biotin per day was enough to make a notable improvement in the firmness and hardness of the nails of individuals who increased their intake of the essential B vitamin over a five-month period.

Other Essential Nutrients

Have you ever heard the expression that healthy people seem to "glow"? The truth is that your skin is the outer reflection of your internal health—so eating a diet that is rich in antioxidants and that otherwise promotes good health will naturally have you *looking* as good as you feel.

ESSENTIAL

Brazil nuts are a wonderful food for skin health. Why? Because Brazil nuts are high in selenium. Selenium has been shown to improve skin elasticity, help to combat skin infections, and may even help decrease outbreaks of acne. Selenium is also a key part of the body's production of glutathione, which attacks free radicals in the body that can lead to the deterioration of collagen and elastin in the skin. Selenium also improves the health and appearance of hair and nails.

Minerals as well as vitamins play a role in keeping skin healthy and preventing typical skin issues. Selenium, for example, has been shown to increase the skin's ability to protect you from UV rays and can help reduce sunburns. Copper and zinc, much like vitamin C, help to provide a greater production of, and strengthening of, elastin. Elastin is the fibers that support the skin from underneath. Weak elastin is one of the primary causes of sagging skin and wrinkles.

DMAE

Dimethylaminoethanol (DMAE) is a powerful antioxidant with many health benefits. DMAE is found in food sources such as sardines, anchovies, and other "oily fish." DMAE has a huge appetite for the free radicals that damage skin. Another is alpha lipoic acid. Alpha lipoic acid is a great antioxidant for skin health because it is one of the few antioxidants that can penetrate both oil and water, meaning it can help both on and below the surface of the skin.

Vitamin A

A skin healthy diet can keep anyone's skin and nails looking their very best at any age and any time of the year. However, sometimes there are chronic skin conditions that cause suffering and can be embarrassing, inconvenient, and sometimes quite painful. Psoriasis is one of these, and recent studies have found that there are nutritional ways to lessen the flare up of psoriasis issues. Vitamin A is a powerful antioxidant, and critical to overall skin health. A recent study published in the *British Journal of Dermatology*, found that foods high in beta-carotene—a form of vitamin A—seems to lessen the symptoms of psoriasis.

Omega-3s

Acne, too, is a skin issue that many have had to "face" at one time or another. Adjusting the diet can also lessen outbreaks and the severity of blackheads, whiteheads, and pimples. Food nutrients good for general skin health have a great impact on lessening acne outbreaks as well. These nutrients include the catechins found in green tea, omega-3 fish oils, and the phytochemicals found in berries. Of course, acne eruptions can be minimized by avoiding some of the known facial irritants such as fast foods, processed foods, and other foods loaded with bad fats.

FACT

Phytonutrients are known for their powerful antioxidant effects. The phytonutrients known as catechins, which are found in green tea, have been shown in clinical studies to help prevent the breakdown of collagen, and therefore green tea should be part of any skin healthy diet.

Other Antioxidants

Varicose veins are not pretty and can be debilitating. A diet rich in the antioxidants described here can also help to lessen the appearance of varicose and spider veins. A compound called *aescin*, found in chestnuts, has been found to strengthen the walls of veins and to minimize the issues of varicose veins. The bromelain in pineapples has been reported to have a similar effect, as well as the nutrient quercetin, found in onions.

You can do your best to keep yourself feeling young and looking young by eating right, being positive and optimistic, and taking the best care that you can of the skin that you are in!

What to Put in Your Shopping Cart

Here are some of the foods that contain the wonderful nutrients that can help you with your cleanse, as well as your healthy daily life. Choose as many as you can, and continue to choose them even after your cleanse.

- **Vitamin A foods:** dark green leafy vegetables such as spinach and kale, broccoli, sweet potatoes, and dairy
- **Vitamin B complex foods (biotin):** peanuts, almonds, lentils, bananas, eggs, oatmeal, and rice
- **Other B vitamin foods:** milk, poultry, oily fish, wheat germ, soybeans, bell peppers, spinach, garlic, celery, cremini mushrooms, and sweet potatoes
- **Vitamin C foods:** citrus fruits such as oranges, grapefruits, lemons, cantaloupe, bell peppers, broccoli, cauliflower, leafy greens, and sweet potatoes
- **Vitamin E foods:** nuts, seeds, olives, egg yolks, soybeans, and wheat germ
- **Zinc foods:** oysters, seafood, lean meat, poultry, and lentils
- **Selenium foods:** whole-grain breads and cereals, seafood, garlic, eggs, nuts, mushrooms, and beans
- **Omega-3 foods:** cold-water fish, including salmon, sardines, and mackerel, flaxseed, flax and safflower oil, nuts, and walnuts
- **Iron foods:** whole grains, leafy greens, liver, prunes, wheat germ, and pumpkin seeds
- **Antioxidant foods:** berries, plums, cantaloupe, artichokes, beans, and pecans
- **Polyphenol foods:** green tea
- **Acidophilus foods:** yogurt

How a Cleanse Can Help

It's easy to shower or bathe and shampoo as often as you like, and it seems with lather and soap and sponges, and whatever products you use, the cleansing process should take care of your skin, hair, and nails, leaving you squeaky clean, fresh, and glowing. But sadly, it doesn't always seem to work—because what is really needed are important changes on the inside. Doing a cleanse for clearer skin and stronger nails will be a start to filling your body with the nutrients that your skin needs to be healthy.

ESSENTIAL

Amino acids are essential for the formation of all types of collagen. There are different collagen types, each with a particular degree of strength and flexibility. A good source of one of these collagen-building amino acids, proline, is an egg white.

Plan to do your cleanse for one to three days. Begin your cleanse in the morning with a large glass of water with a squirt of lemon or lime juice and 1–2 teaspoons of ground flaxseed. Choose a fruit-based beverage for breakfast, and either a vegetable soup or beverage for lunch and dinner. Following are some suggested recipes.

Imbibe water and green and herbal teas liberally throughout the day. For snacks, here are a few suggestions: a blended mixture of a ½ cup of fat-free yogurt with ½ cucumber, a sprig of dill, water and ice; a blended mixture of ½ cup fat-free yogurt with 1 ounce soaked almonds, 1 cup water, ice, 1 pitted date or dry prune, and ½ teaspoon cinnamon; a blended drink of ¼–½ cup watermelon with 1 cup of water, a mint leave (optional), and ice; or a clear broth.

After the Cleanse

Following your cleanse, here are some things to keep in mind:

- Begin to increase your selection and amounts of solid foods. A great interim meal suggestion is to spread a slice of whole-grain pita with

1 tablespoon of hummus, and top with ½ can of mashed sardines in olive oil or tomato sauce.
- Always make sure your system has important probiotics and prebiotics. Dairy sources include yogurt, kefir, and cottage cheese. Nondairy sources include tofu, soy yogurt, miso, tempeh, and sauerkraut.
- Keep your drinking/flushing habits alive with herbal teas and water.
- Do some exercise—both cardio and strength training. Aim for four times a week, and walk every day. Dermatologists recommend exercise as a means to a better complexion. Exercise can even control breakouts, because sweating can help unclog pores. Exercise reduces stress, which tends to lessen hormone output, which can help control skin flare-ups—and is even good for hair.
- Stretching is important. It increases oxygen and blood flow, and decreases stress.

Remember that there are many, many wonderful and nutritious foods you can choose from that will help your skin to achieve and maintain the clarity you want and keep your nails in top condition. Using a wide variety of foods in your everyday diet is the best way to make the most of what the earth has to offer.

By exercising and making the right food choices you can keep yourself healthy and strong inside and out!

Berry Good for Breakfast Beverage

Leafy greens like kale aren't just for soups and salads; they can bring out the sweetness of fruits like berries and the tartness of dates.

INGREDIENTS | YIELDS 1 SERVING

1 heaping cup chopped fresh kale or spinach leaves

1 cup berries

1–2 pitted prunes or red dates

½–1 banana

2 tablespoons toasted wheat germ

1 cup water

1 cup soy, skim, rice, or almond milk

Cinnamon, to taste (optional)

Stevia, to taste (optional)

2–3 ice cubes, for desired amount of "iciness"

Combine all the ingredients in a blender and blend until smooth. Pour into a glass and serve.

Green but Not Martian Beverage

Nuts like almonds, cashews, and walnuts are referred to as "brain foods" because they contain high levels of omega-3s, which are believed to enhance brain power and critical thinking.

INGREDIENTS | YIELDS 1 SERVING

1 orange, cut into sections

½ banana

1 cup fresh chopped Swiss chard, kale, collard greens, or spinach

1–2 pitted prunes or red dates

½ cup ground cashews, walnuts, or almonds (soaked in water for a few hours to soften for easy blending)

2 tablespoons toasted wheat germ

1½ cups water

1 (2-ounce) scoop whey or soy protein powder

1–2 teaspoons ground flaxseed

2–3 ice cubes, if desired for "iciness" level

Combine all the ingredients in a blender and blend until smooth. Pour into a glass and serve.

Shiitake Mushroom Barley Soup

This soup, which is excellent for skin, was created and suggested by Gayle Stolove, BS, RN, LMT, macrobiotic educator, personal chef, and founder of Wholly Macro, www.whollymacrobiotics.com.

INGREDIENTS | YIELDS 4–5 SERVINGS

¼ cup whole barley

¼ cup pearled barley

3 cups spring water

3 dried shiitake mushrooms, soaked in ½ cup water until tender, then sliced

½ yellow onion, cut into medium dice

1 stalk celery, cut into medium dice

2 carrots, cut into short, thin matchsticks

1 tablespoon low-sodium soy sauce

Sprig of fresh dill or parsley, minced

Pearls of Beauty

This delicious soup is a rich and creamy blend of high-fiber whole-grain barley and pearled barley. In Eastern medicine, various types of barley are known as pearls of beauty, and are prized for their ability to restore the skin to flawless, creamy perfection. This humble grain cleanses the blood of accumulated fat and waste debris that can make the skin look lifeless and washed out.

1. Rinse both barleys until the rinse water is clear (3 or 4 times) and dispose of water.

2. Place the soaked barley in a saucepan. Add the 3 cups spring water. Cover and cook over low to medium heat for at least 1 hour, until the barley is soft and creamy.

3. Add the shiitake mushrooms and their soaking water and cook for another 15 minutes.

4. Add the onions and cook for another 15 minutes.

5. Add the carrots and cook for 15 more minutes.

6. Turn down heat, add the celery and soy sauce, and simmer for 5 minutes, then turn off heat. Let sit for at least 15 more minutes, uncovered.

7. Carefully place the mixture in the blender, including the parsley, blend until smooth and serve warm.

Spinach Soup Skinsational

Spinach is a great source of nutrients for skin and nail issues, and coupled with tasty ingredients like garlic and lemon juice, you won't even know you're drinking a veggie!

INGREDIENTS | YIELDS 1–2 SERVINGS

2 cups fresh spinach, chopped fine

½ cup finely chopped onion

1 clove finely minced garlic

2½ cups vegetable or chicken broth

1 teaspoon fresh lemon juice

1 tablespoon extra-virgin olive oil

1 egg

½ cup cashews, soaked in water to soften for easy blending

Sea salt and ground black pepper, to taste

1–2 tablespoons nonfat, plain Greek-style yogurt (optional)

1. In a pot over medium-low heat, cook the spinach, cashews, onion, garlic, broth, lemon juice, and oil for 15 minutes.

2. In a small bowl, beat the egg by hand. Add a little hot soup to the egg and mix. Add the egg mixture to the pot of soup, stirring constantly for 4 minutes more. Let cool a little.

3. Carefully add the soup mixture to a blender and blend (being careful the hot soup does not splash out). Can be served warm or cold with a dollop of yogurt.

Chickpea Vegetable Soup

Chickpeas, which really look like little beans, are used as main ingredients in such foods as hummus and falafel.

INGREDIENTS | YIELDS 2–3 SERVINGS

1 small onion, peeled and diced

1 carrot, scrubbed and diced

1 red bell pepper, chopped

2 stalks celery, diced

1 clove garlic, minced

1 tablespoon extra-virgin olive oil

4 cups vegetable broth

1 (6-ounce) can chickpeas drained

1 small sweet potato, peeled and diced

⅓ cup cashews, soaked in water to soften

½ teaspoon optional seasonings: cumin, coriander, salt, pepper

1 teaspoon lemon or orange juice

1. In a large pot, sauté the onion, carrot, bell pepper, celery, and garlic in the oil until tender.

2. Add the broth, chickpeas, sweet potato, and cashews. Add seasonings to taste. Simmer until tender, about 10 minutes.

3. Remove from heat and allow to cool a little. Add to a blender and purée. Stir in the lemon or orange juice.

CHAPTER 8

Cleansing for a Detoxed Filtering System

Everyone has probably had the experience, at least once, of having to find a rest room, especially following several cups of coffee, or of not being able to find a restroom as quickly as one would wish. The truth is that it really is necessary to use rest rooms frequently, and to keep healthy amounts of fluids washing through your body. But sometimes you may be avoiding the "nuisance" of a rest stop, or even avoiding voiding urine because of discomfort or pain. Helping your body's filtering system work smoothly and frequently is an important function of cleansing.

Typical Kidney Issues

If you are holding up your natural irrigation system because it might be painful to go, or you just don't have the time to "get up and go," you are preventing your body's natural filtering system from working properly and allowing waste and toxins to accumulate.

ESSENTIAL

Water is essential to overall health, and of course good kidney function. You are probably familiar with the 8/8 rule: 8 glasses of 8 ounces of water per day as a guideline. Some health care practitioners recommend drinking the equivalent of half your body weight in ounces of water per day to avoid such problems. For example, if you weigh 160 pounds, then you should drink at least 80 ounces of water, which is equivalent to approximately ten 8-ounce glasses.

Just the way you cleanse anything by washing, the kidneys filter your system in a washing process. You need healthy functioning kidneys to be able to keep your body cleanly flushed and detoxed. You need that fluid, especially water, irrigating and filtering your body.

Get Enough H$_2$0

It happens in the day to day that many people don't have the time to drink enough cleansing water. Who wants to think about drinking all the time—with the inconvenience of "pit stops" or when meetings are scheduled, or rush-hour traffic is reckoned with. This all does not do your body's irrigation system justice. Plants need enough water to thrive, and so does your kidney system.

ALERT

Don't "hold it in." It is never a good idea to fight the urge to urinate. The kidneys can only hold so much water. Always relieve yourself when you feel you have to. Kidney cells are elastic, but holding it too long can cause damage.

Every day your kidneys have to process, or filter, the waste out of close to 200 quarts of blood. From that, on average about 2 quarts are passed per day as urine. As you might imagine, that requires a lot of "plumbing," and there are several areas along the way where problems can happen. Besides filtering waste products and keeping the blood clean and healthy, the kidneys also make various hormones, regulate the pH balance of the blood-stream, and help to keep up the needed amounts of blood plasma.

Minor kidney dysfunction can lead to poor health; major kidney dysfunction can be fatal. But even serious conditions such as chronic kidney disease may be avoided with a more kidney healthy diet. In fact, many health care professionals agree that poor diet is the single greatest contributing factor to kidney problems.

Chronic Kidney Disease and Other Infections

Often it is other things that lead to serious or chronic kidney disease, the two most likely culprits being diabetes and high blood pressure—both of which are also complications of poor diets and obesity. Chronic kidney disease is a serious medical condition, often needing dialysis, a process in which a machine is used as a substitute for the normal filtering of the kidneys.

ALERT

According to the National Institutes of Health, chronic kidney disease (CKD) is reaching epidemic proportions, with as many as 26 million Americans suffering from some form of kidney disease. The high amount of toxins in the environment and food supply that is causing the kidneys to work harder has been noted as a reason for the huge increase.

Other than chronic kidney disease, the two most common and less life threatening problems with the kidneys are infections and blockages. Bacterial infection can cause inflammation of the kidneys. Though not a kidney issue per se, urinary tract infections and bladder infections are also common problems related to the elimination of liquid waste. In fact, almost all bacterial infections of the kidneys start out as urinary tract infections (UTI) and/or bladder infections, which then travel to the kidneys. UTIs and bladder infections can also be avoided or lessened with a kidney healthy diet.

The other common issues related to kidneys are blockages, such as kidney stones, which get in the way of the flow of waste from the kidneys. A kidney stone is a hard mass that forms from crystals that separate out from urine in the urinary tract. Most times if such crystals form, they are still tiny enough to pass through the urinary tract and out of the body without any issues. However, sometimes they become too large, and a kidney stone is the result. Kidney stones can be very painful. If left untreated they can lead to serious complications. Often, stones can "pass" on their own; other times medical intervention is needed to break up or dissolve the stone.

ALERT

Kidney trouble? Your body has several ways of letting you know. Symptoms of a kidney disorder can be dizziness, headache, puffiness around the eyes, edema (swelling), nausea, darkening of the finger nails, dry mouth, thirst, increased need to urinate or difficulty urinating, or severe pain in back or legs.

Certainly there are these specific kidney and urinary issues such as stones and infections that a kidney healthy diet can help to avoid. However, because of the important role the kidneys have in the body, poor kidney function makes a big difference to overall heath. Kidneys with issues can lead to other conditions not necessarily labeled as "kidney disease," such as heart disease, stroke, or even cancer.

Best Nutrients for Good Kidney Function

You know those additives that are put into gasoline, enzymes and other mysterious ingredients that they say boost your car's performance between tune-ups by cleaning out the fuel injectors and other gunk and deposits in your engine? Well, eating the right nutrients is like the "between tune-ups tune-up" for your kidneys. These nutrients all have been shown to enhance kidney function and keep your body's filtration system running smoothly and efficiently.

Get Your Bs

As you might imagine, vitamins and antioxidants are on the frontline in good kidney health. B vitamins, especially the B_6 pyridoxamine, have been shown to actually limit the buildup of what are called *glycation end products* (AGEs) in the kidneys. AGEs have been found to be a precursor to chronic kidney disease. Vitamin B_2 also has been shown to have a positive effect on kidney function, as have vitamins E and C.

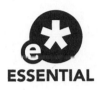

ESSENTIAL

B vitamins are essential to kidney health, but cooking and processing decreases the level of Bs in many foods containing them. Vegetables lose approximately 60–80 percent of their B_6 when canned, fruits about 38 percent, both fruits and veggies lose about 15 percent when frozen, and grains lose about 50–95 percent of their level of B_6 when they are converted from whole grains to grain products.

Antioxidants

Because of the huge amounts of toxins that pass through the kidneys daily, they are, with the exception of the liver, the organs in the body that get the greatest amount of oxidative stress and possible damage by free radicals. CoQ10, with its clinically proven and powerful antioxidant action, is so important to support good kidney health. Silymarin, a flavonoid and strong antioxidant found in milk thistle, has also been shown in clinical studies to target free-radical attack on the kidneys. Research seems to point out that silymarin can be effective in removing toxins from medications that the kidneys are not always able to remove and eliminate as waste.

Resveratrol, found in red wine and dark-colored berries, is considered a super-antioxidant. Resveratrol has been shown to effectively lessen the risk of heart disease, and recent evidence suggests it may have a similar effect in lowering the risk of kidney disease as well. Like silymarin, resveratrol's powerful anti-inflammatory and antioxidant action is also believed to combat kidney damage resulting from certain medications.

Lipoic and Amino Acids

Like resveratrol and CoQ10, lipoic acid is another powerful antioxidant with many benefits, including improved kidney function. Lipoic acid is good for general kidney health, and it seems to be helpful in lowering the chances of kidney problems that can result from diabetes.

ESSENTIAL

Celery seeds have been shown to help to increase the kidneys ability to eliminate water and fluids from the joints, and so can be helpful with many forms of edema (swelling) such as that which is caused by arthritis.

Not having enough of the amino acid carnitine is a known cause of kidney disease, and the amino acid L-carnitine is essential to a kidney healthy diet. It has also been found that most often people with chronic kidney disease, especially those who require dialysis, develop a carnitine deficiency.

A diet that is friendly to your kidneys will have all of the above nutrients, in addition to these others you may already know about: omega-3s and folic acid.

Out with the Bad, In with the Good

A discussion about what nutrients you should include in your diet for good kidney health would not be complete without some talk about what to take out or decrease: bad fats, processed foods, and salt. Excess salt intake has been linked to hypertension, or high blood pressure, which is one of the leading causes of kidney disease. Not only that, but too much salt in the kidneys also limits their ability to filter wastes properly. Buildup of salts in the kidney is one of the most common reasons for edema—or so-called fluid retention.

A low-salt diet helps to prevent or control high blood pressure, as does increasing certain vitamins and nutrients, such as vitamin D.

Berry Berry Yummy!

It has long been known that cranberries really help urinary health and can prevent urinary tract infections (UTIs). A scientific basis has been found for this well-known "folk remedy." Cranberries, more specifically cranberry juice, increase the acidity of urine, which makes it hard for bacteria to live. It also contains an antibacterial agent called *hippuric acid* and other substances that actually prevent E. coli bacteria—which are the cause of UTIs—from sticking to the lining of the urinary tract. These substances are also in blueberries, but not as powerful. However, because of blueberries' additional antioxidant punch, blueberries should also be part of your kidney healthy diet.

FACT

Vitamin D is not only an essential nutrient for good kidney health, but it has also been shown to prevent the onset of flu—even the H1N1, or swine flu. Milk, eggs, and cod liver oil are excellent sources of vitamin D.

Cranberries, blueberries, and their cousin bilberries all also contain quinic acid, which helps to break down calcium and helps to prevent calcified substances from binding together. This means that not only are they recommended to prevent UTIs, but also kidney stones, another common kidney problem. The magnesium and potassium in cranberries also helps to prevent stones from forming by helping to eliminate calcium deposits in the blood. Note these recommendations are to prevent the formation of the most common form of kidney stones—calcium oxide stones, which form when calcium is not removed effectively from the bloodstream. Another type of kidney stone, uric acid stones, are the result of the medical condition gout. If you already have stones, it is important that a medical diagnosis of the type of stones is made. Increased consumption of cranberry juice is not recommended for those with uric acid stones, as it can actually increase their formation.

What to Put in Your Shopping Cart

Here are some of the foods that are rich in nutrients that can help you in your cleanse, as well as help your body anytime. Use as many of them as you wish during your cleanse, and choose them often for your regular daily diet.

- **Foods with vitamin B:** spinach, bell peppers, turnip greens, garlic, cauliflower, celery, cabbage, asparagus, mushrooms, broccoli, collard greens, Brussels sprouts, turmeric, tuna, cod, salmon, snapper, halibut, chicken, calf liver, and turkey
- **Foods with vitamin C:** citrus fruits, strawberry, papaya, cantaloupe, raspberry, watermelon, pineapple, parsley, broccoli, bell peppers, cauliflower, mustard greens, kiwis, snow peas, and zucchini
- **Foods with vitamin D:** salmon, sardines, shrimp, milk, cod, and eggs
- **Foods with vitamin E:** mustard greens, Swiss chard, spinach, olives, turnip greens, sunflower seeds, almonds, papaya, and blueberries
- **Foods with CoQ10:** fish, liver, heart, kidney, wheat germ, and whole grains
- **Foods with lipoic acid:** broccoli, spinach, collard greens, Swiss chard, calf liver, round steak, and brewer's yeast
- **Foods with carnitine:** beef, milk, codfish, chicken, and Cheddar cheese
- **Foods with potassium:** cabbage, tomatoes, cantaloupe, lima beans, avocados, cucumber, celery, kale, soybeans, and seeds
- **Foods with magnesium:** Swiss chard, spinach, yellow squash, broccoli, mustard greens, and dried basil
- **Foods with silymarin:** milk thistle tea, artichokes, turmeric, and coriander
- **Foods with resveratrol:** red grapes, wine, grape juice, peanuts, blueberries, and bilberries

How a Cleanse Can Help

Your kidneys are your body's main filtration system. Now, if you ever have had to change the filter on your air conditioner, your water tap, or the air filter in your car, then one thing you know about filters is that they get clogged up and need to be changed often to keep working properly. Well, you really can't change the filters on your kidneys, but you can give them a good jump-start to cleaner health with a nutritional cleanse. Using proper nutrition in your selection of foods and beverages can really make a difference to your kidneys and help to ward off some of those uncomfortable issues.

ESSENTIAL

Since alcohol is a diuretic (increases the need to urinate), you might think drinking alcoholic beverages is good for your kidneys. But not so. Drink in moderation; those extra cocktails may make you hit the restroom at the bar more often, but they make your kidneys work overtime to remove the other messes that alcohol can leave behind. Alcohol actually prevents the elimination of uric acid. Buildup of uric acid can cause gout and kidney stones.

Plan to do your cleanse from one to three days. Begin your day with 12–16 ounces of water with a squirt of lemon or lime juice and a teaspoon of ground flaxseed. One of your main goals is to get your kidneys accustomed to water all the time—no more thirst issues that promote kidney issues. Choose a breakfast, lunch, and dinner, and two snacks between the meals. Following are some suggested recipes.

For your snacks, you could choose a blended drink of 1 celery stalk, 1 cucumber, 1 cut-up orange, a small piece of fresh ginger, and water. An excellent drink for kidneys recommended by macrobiotic educators is watermelon and water. Use the white area of the watermelon as well, and blend it in a blender, along with a squeeze of lemon or lime juice. Make sure to drink your fluids every hour, including water, and herbal teas. Of course, a handful of cranberries or a little pure cranberry juice is supreme, combined with a few strawberries, red grapes, water, and ice.

After the Cleanse

Following your cleanse, here are some things to keep in mind:

- Begin to increase your selection and amounts of solid foods. A great interim meal suggestion is to spread a slice of whole-grain pita with 1 tablespoon of hummus, and top with a ½ small can of mashed salmon, tuna in water, or herring with a slice of tomato.
- Always make sure your system has important probiotics and pre-biotics. Dairy sources include yogurt, kefir, and cottage cheese. Nondairy sources include tofu, soy yogurt, miso, tempeh, and sauerkraut.
- Keep your drinking/flushing habits alive with herbal teas and water. Enjoy your cranberry juice.
- Do some exercise—both cardio and strength training. Aim for four times a week, and walk every day.
- Stretching is important. It increases oxygen and blood flow, and decreases stress.

ALERT

Salad in general, eaten at least once a day, has been shown to decrease the risk of kidney cancer by as much as 40 percent. Root vegetables and white cabbage offer the most protection, providing a 50–65 percent decrease in risk.

Fiber is crucial in a healthy diet for kidney health, and it has other health benefits as well. Evidence has shown that people using processed food that does not contain fiber are among those who fall into kidney problems. Fruits, vegetables, nuts, and whole grains are excellent sources.

Remember that there are many, many wonderful and nutritious foods you can choose from that will help your kidneys to be in the best of health and the rest of your body too. Using a wide variety of foods in your everyday diet is the way to make the most of what the earth has to offer. By making the right food choices your kidneys will thank you, and you'll keep your internal plumbing working properly.

Azuki Bean Attitude for Kidney

This soup, a favorite for kidney cleanse and any time, was recommended and created by Gayle Stolove, BS, RN, LMT, macrobiotic educator, personal chef, and founder of Wholly Macro, www.whollymacrobiotics.com.

INGREDIENTS | YIELDS 4–6 SERVINGS

2 cups dry azuki beans

8 cups spring water, divided

1 teaspoon sea salt

1 tablespoon barley malt or honey

½ cup chopped fresh chives

1 tablespoon sesame oil

1 medium-sized yellow onion, diced

1 tablespoon fresh ginger, grated

1 cup chopped carrot or butternut squash

Bean There, Done That!

The liquid left over from the cooked azuki beans is called Azuki Bean Tea, and can be taken fresh as a warm tea, as a kidney and adrenal tonic to warm and strengthen weak kidneys and exhausted adrenals. Deep red azuki beans are traditionally known in Eastern medicine to strengthen and vitalize the kidneys and adrenals. They are also high in essential bone-strengthening minerals.

1. In advance, rinse the azuki beans 2–3 times, until the rinse water is clear, and then soak the beans in 4 cups of spring water for at least 2 hours, or overnight.

2. Drain the beans, but reserve the soaking water for tea (see the sidebar below).

3. Cook the azuki beans in the 4 cups water, bringing the water to a simmer; skim off and discard the foam as it forms at the top, using a small strainer. After the foam stops forming, cover and simmer for 40 minutes, or until the beans are soft.

4. Add the salt, barley malt or honey, and chives, and cook an additional 15 minutes.

5. Add the sesame oil to a frying pan over medium heat. Add the onion and ginger and sauté until tender about 3–4 minutes. Then add the carrot or squash and sauté until tender, about 10–15 minutes.

6. Combine the beans and vegetables and carefully pour into blender in batches and blend until smooth. Serve warm.

Yellow—A Great Color for Squash Soup

This mixture is such a friendly color, you'll want to have it on cold winter afternoons to warm you up.

INGREDIENTS | YIELDS 2 SERVINGS

2 cups chopped yellow summer squash

1 cup frozen green peas

½ cup chopped carrot

½ cup chopped celery

½–1 clove minced garlic

½ teaspoon dried dill

2 cups low or no-salt chicken or vegetable broth

½ cup water

¼ cup nonfat, plain Greek-style yogurt (optional)

1. In a large pot, combine all the ingredients except the yogurt. Simmer for 15 minutes.

2. Pour into a blender in batches (being careful not to splash it and burn yourself) and blend until smooth.

3. Stir in the yogurt if desired. May be chilled for 1 hour and served cold as well.

Cabbage Capital Anytime Soup

*Cabbage is a great cleanser for your kidneys, and as a leafy green,
chock-full of the nutrients your body needs to keep the system flushed.*

INGREDIENTS | YIELDS 4 SERVINGS

2 cups water

3 cups shredded cabbage (about 1 pound)

1 cup chopped onion

1 cup diced, peeled beets

¼ cup chopped celery

½ cup chopped carrots

1 cup diced tomatoes

¼ cup raisins

½ cup frozen lima beans

¼ cup tomato sauce

Fresh lemon juice, to taste

Sea salt and pepper, to taste

2 tablespoons–¼ cup nonfat, plain Greek-style yogurt or soy yogurt (optional)

1. In a large pot, combine the water, cabbage, onion, beets, celery, carrots, tomatoes, raisins, lima beans, and tomato sauce. Bring to a boil.

2. Cover and simmer 1 hour.

3. Carefully blend the ingredients, adding lemon juice, salt, and pepper to taste, and additional water if necessary. Mix in yogurt to taste, if desired, and serve.

A Cranberry Blender Booster

Cranberries have a powerful, healing effect on your kidneys. Often used as a home remedy to treat urinary tract infections, cranberry juice is a delicious alternative to antibiotics.

INGREDIENTS | YIELDS 1 SERVING

½ cup cranberry juice (100% juice, no corn syrup added)

½ cup blueberries

1 (2-ounce) scoop whey or soy protein powder

½ cup soy or fat-free milk

¼ cup egg substitute

1 cup water

2 tablespoons wheat germ

1–2 teaspoons stevia, if desired

2–3 ice cubes, or to taste for desired "iciness"

Combine all the ingredients in a blender and blend until smooth. Pour into a glass and serve.

Creamy Fruit and Veggie Mix and Match

This recipe combines fruits and a great green to create a delicious mixture that will jump-start your kidneys—makes you think fruits and veggies should pair up more often!

INGREDIENTS | YIELDS 1 SERVING

1 cup soy, rice, or almond milk

1 cup water

½ banana

¾–1 cup berries, pears, or cantaloupe

2 tablespoons toasted wheat germ

1 dried, pitted date or prune

1 cup chopped kale

1 (2-ounce) scoop whey or soy protein powder

Cinnamon, to taste (optional)

2–3 ice cubes for desired level of "iciness" (optional)

1 teaspoon stevia (optional)

1 teaspoon ground flaxseed

Combine all the ingredients in a blender and blend until smooth.

CHAPTER 9

Cleansing for a Healthy Heart

Often the things the news reports say to worry about when it comes to your heart are shrouded in a haze of numbers and statistics. But, it is good to note that research and science has definite facts and figures on keeping your heart strong, nutrition that contributes to heart health, and guidelines that you should know about.

Typical Heart and Circulatory Issues

Do you like your foods to leave an oily coating on your lips? Do you like to shake the salt on everything? Do you frequent fast-food restaurants? Do you like your treats and sweets often as rewards? If so, you may not be doing your heart any good.

FACT

A study found that men in Greece have a genetic predisposition to high cholesterol, and yet the population overall has a low amount of heart disease. The reason? Many scientists believe it is the use of olive oil in the diet. The good monounsaturated fats in olive oil lowers "bad" LDL cholesterol and reduces the risk of heart disease. Look for the least-processed olive oils—the extra-virgin or virgin varieties—and use it instead of butter or other oils when cooking.

Your heart is like the royal queen and king sitting at the center throne of the body, and it has many passions in nutrients. And if it isn't getting these it can be dethroned and maybe not even tell you about it until it just quits, taking *you* with it! So, now is really the time to get to the heart of the matter of a healthy heart.

Cardiovascular Disease

A healthy heart is key to maintaining strength, stamina, and fitness. A healthy heart means you will live longer. But, when anyone talks about keeping the heart strong and healthy the biggest concern is really the prevention of the number one killer in the United States: cardiovascular disease (CVD). Most often when people think of cardiovascular disease they think of strokes and heart attacks. Strokes and heart attacks can be the result of CVD, and often are, but they are not the same things as CVD. In fact, cardiovascular disease itself is not one, but many conditions. But all of these conditions involve a situation when the crucial vessels of the circulatory system cannot do their regular job of getting oxygen and nutrients to and from the vital organs.

Arteriosclerosis and Atherosclerosis

Two conditions of great concern are arteriosclerosis and atherosclerosis. Both involve blockages in the arteries. Arteriosclerosis is most well known as "hardening of the arteries." In arteriosclerosis it is calcified deposits called *plaque* that form the blockages and stop blood flow. When this happens in the arteries that bring oxygenated blood to the heart, it is called *coronary artery disease*, or CAD. People with coronary artery disease are at great risk for heart attacks. Atherosclerosis is a similar condition, but the difference is that the blockages are made of fats and lipids, and the arteries usually affected are the carotid arteries.

ALERT

Homocysteine is an amino acid that is a building block of protein, mostly meat protein. High levels of homocysteine in the blood have been linked to a greater possibility for developing coronary artery disease. A higher level of homocysteine in the blood is often caused by a vitamin B deficiency; increased intake of foods rich in vitamin B may help to control the levels of homocysteine in the blood.

The carotid arteries bring oxygenated blood to the brain, and therefore people with atherosclerosis are at great risk for strokes. Both conditions are severely impacted by diet. The typical high-fat, high-cholesterol diet of many Americans is the leading cause of both conditions. It is not unusual for people who eat a diet of mostly fast food, processed foods, and red meats, to be at risk for developing both conditions.

People with CVD, especially with coronary artery disease, are also likely to develop hypertension or high blood pressure. This is because the blood has to work harder to push through the narrowed vessels. High blood pressure also increases the risk of heart attack and stroke, as well as kidney disease.

Arrhythmia

Coronary artery disease is one of the most common heart-related issues, and should be of serious concern to those at risk. Other heart issues include arrhythmia, which is an abnormal heart rhythm, problems with one or more of the heart valves, cardiomyopathy, which is a thickening of the heart muscle, and congestive heart failure.

ESSENTIAL

Avocados are an excellent source of heart healthy fats. Avocados are loaded with monounsaturated fat and have been shown to help lower LDL ("bad") cholesterol levels while raising HDL ("good") cholesterol levels.

Basically, the heart is a pump. Picture a mountain with a water pump at the base with tubes that bring water from a lake nearby for irrigating all the plants around the mountain. The heart is like that pump, and the arteries are the irrigation tubes, bringing blood to the organs. If there's a clog in the tube you can see there could be a bad problem. This is really what happens in CAD. Another thing that could happen on that mountain is the tubes could be okay, but the pump begins to get weak, and then the water doesn't get pumped as well as it should. The plants farthest away from the pump would weaken and die, and the water in the lake behind the pump would start to accumulate and back up because it is no longer being normally circulated around the mountain.

Congestive Heart Failure

Congestive heart failure (CHF)—commonly referred to simply as heart failure, or as a "weak heart"—and CAD are closely related. Anything that causes the heart to work harder can eventually cause it to weaken, so coronary artery disease can be a cause of congestive heart failure. Problems that can be a part of a weakened heart that is trying to work harder are swelling of the legs and ankles, fatigue, shortness of breath, and overall weakness.

Best Nutrients for Heart Health

Study after study that compares rates of heart disease worldwide have found that the United States has a higher incidence of heart disease than most other countries, and the reason stated is diet. One such study in particular tracked the diets of 16,000 middle-aged men from the United States, Finland, the Netherlands, Italy, Greece, and Japan for a period of twenty-five years. When the typical food patterns were analyzed cross-culturally it was found that in countries such as Japan and Greece, where there was a higher consumption of vegetables, legumes, fish, and whole-grain cereals, rather than the typical red meat diet of the men in the United States, the risk of death from heart disease dropped a whopping 82 percent.

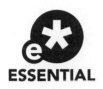

ESSENTIAL

Heart healthy entrées should have no more than 3 grams of saturated fat, unless the main course is fish. Fish entrées can have up to 5 grams of saturated fats, since the added benefits of omega-3 fish oils out weigh the downside of the extra saturated fats.

Fiber Again

Fiber has long been linked to lowering the risk of heart disease. This is because fiber, especially the fiber in whole grains, has been shown to lower LDL, the so-called bad cholesterol that is a leading cause of coronary artery disease. Whole-grain fiber also has a powerful antioxidant effect, which protects the heart and its valves and arteries from oxidative stress and free-radical damage. For example, wheat bran has twenty times the antioxidative power of refined white flour. Whole grains also contain phytoestrogens, the same plant compounds that are also in soy that give soy and soy products their ability to lower bad cholesterol levels. Whole grains also contain other cholesterol fighting nutrients such as plant sterols, stanols, and saponins.

Magnesium and Folate

Many of the foods in heart-healthy diets also have high levels of magnesium and folate, both of which also help to cleanse the blood of cholesterol and other elements, specifically calcium, which can form plaque buildup in the arteries. Magnesium and folate have also been found to prevent free-radical damage to the heart.

The spice turmeric, the key ingredient in curry, is also very high in both magnesium and folate. Compared to the United States, rates of heart disease in India are far lower. The flavonoid curcuma is believed to be the reason for turmeric's heart healthy actions. Curcuma is also found in garlic and onions, so while a nice meal of sautéed onions and garlic may keep some friends and the occasional vampire away, it will also fend off heart disease.

FACT

Many people think that Quinoa is a grain, but it is actually a tiny sprouted seed. An excellent source of magnesium, this mineral lowers cholesterol, making it a good choice to include in a heart-healthy diet.

Red Wine

In general, use of alcoholic beverages in excess is not good for the heart, or any other major organ of the body for that matter. However, red wine in moderation can help to prevent heart disease. This is because of the high amount of powerful flavonoids, specifically resveratrol, found in red wine. In fact, resveratrol, a powerful antioxidant with many nutritional benefits, first came to light as being responsible for the so-called "French paradox"—the relatively low number of heart disease among the French population, even though the traditional French diet was high in fat.

Other Nutrients That Promote Heart Health

Other nutrients that should be part of a heart healthy diet are recommended for their powerful antioxidant abilities, which can improve heart strength and function, and/or their proven ability to lower "bad" cholesterol. These include:

- CoQ10
- Omega-3 fatty acids
- Alpha lipoic acids
- L-carnitine
- Vitamin B complex—B_6, B_{12}, and folic acid (B_9)
- Vitamins C and E
- Polyphenols

Chapter 9: Cleansing for a Healthy Heart

- Carotenoids
- Selenium

ESSENTIAL

Hot cocoa is not only a soothing, make you feel all warm inside treat on a cold winter's day—it's also good for your heart! Hot cocoa is packed with antioxidants; in fact, it has twice the antioxidants of red wine and three times as much as are found in green tea. However, pass on the powdered mixes on the supermarket shelves that are filled with added sugar and artificial flavors; instead, use 100 percent cocoa in powdered or bar form—and leave out the sugary mini-marshmallows!

Salt and Your Heart

To be heart healthy there are things you should increase in your diet and things you should decrease or eliminate. When it comes to heart health, the best thing you can do is go to your kitchen table or pantry, grab your saltshaker, and throw it out. Salt, and a high-salt diet, which is typical of the American diet, is a major contributor to high blood pressure and congestive heart failure.

Reducing your salt intake doesn't really mean that you must get rid of that saltshaker altogether, especially if you are a strict vegetarian. But getting label conscious—looking at the sodium content in foods—really helps your salt intake. You will probably be floored at the amounts of sodium found in many canned, frozen, and otherwise processed foods—even in those claiming to be "low-salt." The U.S. recommended daily allowance (RDA) for sodium is 2,300 mg, and 1 teaspoon equals 2,000 mg.

ALERT

Salmon is a fish super-rich in omega-3s, and the carotenoid astaxanthin, a powerful antioxidant. Two to three servings of salmon per week can significantly reduce your risk of heart attack—but choose wild rather than farm-raised salmon. Farm-raised salmon can have unhealthy additives, pesticides, and other toxins.

What to Put in Your Shopping Cart

Here are lists of some foods rich in the nutrients that can help you with your cleanse, and keep your body healthy anytime. Choose and use as many as you can for your cleanse, and in your daily diet afterward.

- **Herbs and spices to replace salt:** basil, marjoram, oregano, parsley, sage, thyme, rosemary, dill weed, cinnamon, chili powder, cloves, ginger, nutmeg, curry, cumin, coriander, turmeric, and mustard seed
- **Fiber foods:** whole grains, soy, legumes, beans, vegetables, fruits, and wheat germ
- **Vitamin A and carotenoid foods:** citrus fruit, tomatoes, carrots, mango, spinach, and collard greens
- **Vitamin B complex foods:** salmon, tuna, turkey, cod, snapper, halibut, spinach, bell peppers, turnip greens, garlic, cauliflower, celery, cabbage, cremini mushrooms, asparagus, broccoli, collard greens, Brussels sprouts, chard, and turmeric
- **Vitamin C foods:** bell peppers, parsley, broccoli, peppers, berries, citrus fruits, papaya, cauliflower, mustard greens, spinach, snow peas, cantaloupe, watermelon, tomato, zucchini, and celery
- **Vitamin E foods:** mustard greens, chard, turnip greens, almonds, spinach, sunflower seeds, olives, papaya, and blueberries
- **Magnesium and folate foods:** beans, turmeric, spinach, squash, and mustard greens
- **Flavonoid foods:** fruits, tea, soy, turnip greens, basil, garlic, onion, red wine, herbs, and spices
- **CoQ10 foods:** fish, wheat germ, and whole grains

- **Omega-3 fatty acid foods:** salmon, flaxseed, walnuts, sardines, soybeans, halibut, tofu, and snapper
- **Lipoic acid foods:** broccoli, spinach, collard greens, Swiss chard, and brewer's yeast
- **Carnitine foods:** codfish, chicken, and beef
- **Polyphenol foods:** green tea, cocoa, apples, citrus fruits, berries, and soy
- **Selenium foods:** Brazil nuts, fish, cremini mushrooms, eggs, lamb, barley, sunflower seeds, turkey, oats, and tofu

How a Cleanse Can Help

As your blood circulates—makes its rounds—and your heart receives the life-giving oxygen it needs, no doubt there have been many things that have entered your body, and some of them may have already done some unhealthy work in your arteries. Here is a chance to put the bad things and lack of good nutrients behind you. Starting off with a cleanse for a healthy heart will keep you beating to a new, healthy drum.

ESSENTIAL

Several studies have strongly indicated that eating 1 ounce of nuts four or five times a week can significantly reduce your risk of coronary artery disease—by as much as 40 percent. The best are almonds, walnuts, macadamia nuts, pecans, and pistachios, all of which are full of omega-3 fatty acids and "good" fats. But go for no-salt or low-salt varieties, pass on honey-roasted or sugar-coated nuts, and remember that all nuts are high in calories, so they should not be added to your diet, but substituted for another source of calories.

Plan to do your cleanse for one to three days. Begin your day with 12–16 ounces of water with a squirt of lemon or lime juice and 1 teaspoon of ground flaxseed. Choose three meals—a nutrient-rich breakfast, lunch, and dinner. In between do drink plenty of herbal teas and water. You may choose some special water beverages by blending a few cubes of watermelon or pineapple and a stalk of celery or cucumber with water and ice. Or, blend a piece of celery, cucumber, orange, and a small piece of fresh ginger with water and ice. Following are some suggested recipes.

After the Cleanse

First, give yourself a star for keeping your heart happily beating into your future. And now you've set a good pattern that really takes care of your blood and how it circulates to your heart.

FACT

High cholesterol is one of the major factors of heart disease. Lowering your cholesterol intake is critical to heart health, but did you know that only 20 percent of your body's cholesterol comes from the food you eat? The other 80 percent is actually manufactured by your liver. There are nutrients, most notability phenols and plant sterols, found naturally in foods that have the same if not better cholesterol-lowering effects as pharmaceuticals, without the side effects. Foods with phenols include olive oil, berries, cherries, plums, and artichokes.

Following your cleanse, here are some things to keep in mind:

- Begin to increase your selection and amounts of solid foods and amounts. A great interim meal suggestion is to spread a slice of whole-grain pita with 1 teaspoon of hummus and ½ can of mashed sardines in olive oil, and top it with slice of tomato.
- Keep your drinking/flushing habits alive with herbal teas and water.
- Do some exercise—both cardio and strength training. Aim for four times a week, and walk every day.
- Stretching is important. It increases oxygen and blood flow, and decreases stress.

Keep some vegetables washed and cut in your refrigerator for quick snacks, and keep fresh fruit out so you don't forget about it. Allow yourself a treat or indulgence from time to time. A candy bar or handful of potato chips isn't going to overthrow a general plan for heart-healthy nutrients in your day to day.

Reduce salt by using herbs and spices. Experiment and try a new one each week. The University of California Medical Center had come up with some lovely recipes for herb and spice mixtures that you can fill a few salt-shakers with. They include:

- 2 tablespoons each of dried basil, marjoram, thyme, rosemary, and red pepper and 1 tablespoon each of garlic powder and dried oregano
- ¼ cup dried parsley, 2 tablespoons dried tarragon, and 1 tablespoon each of dried oregano, dill weed, and celery flakes
- ¼ cup ground ginger, 2 tablespoons each of ground cinnamon and ground cloves, and 1 tablespoon each of ground allspice and anise
- ½ cup dried dill and 1 tablespoon each of dried chives, garlic powder, dried lemon peel, and dried chervil

Plan your meals that will have less sodium. You can do it a little at a time. When you taste your food and you feel the need for salt, try one shake instead of two. When you use canned food, a rinse in water can remove some of the salt.

ESSENTIAL

Get moving! In addition to proper nutrition, one of the best things you can do for heart health is exercise. The American Heart Association recommends at least thirty to sixty minutes of moderate-intensity exercise, at least three to four days a week. What is highly recommended is aerobic, or "cardio," exercises that increase circulation and heart rate, such as walking, running, biking, swimming, etc.

Small things to remember: smoking and secondhand smoke are major causes of heart disease. Try to reduce stress and anxiety; they can lead to high blood pressure and other health conditions. Keep your weight within recommended limits. Obesity is a leading cause of heart disease. A great healthy snack is to make your own trail mix by combining nuts, seeds, dried fruits, and dried oats.

Remember that there are many wonderful and nutritious foods you can choose from that will help your heart to be in the best of health and the rest of your body too. Using a wide variety of foods in your everyday diet is the way to make the most of what the earth has to offer you. If you make the right food choices, your circulation and heart will thank you.

A Corny Squash and Potato Curried Soup

This yummy soup has curry, which is a delicious spice mix that contains a power punch of folate—a great way to stimulate heart health.

INGREDIENTS | YIELDS 3 SERVINGS

½ acorn squash, peeled and cut into cubes

1 sweet potato, peeled and cut into cubes

2 carrots, peeled and cut into medium-sized pieces

½ cup rutabaga, chopped small

½ cup chopped onion

1 chopped apple

1 garlic clove

2 teaspoons extra-virgin olive oil

2 cups sodium-free vegetable or chicken broth

¼ teaspoon sea salt

½ teaspoon turmeric

½ teaspoon curry powder

¼ teaspoon ground cinnamon

Cayenne pepper, to taste (optional)

½ cup frozen corn kernels

½ cup soy milk

1. First sauté the onion and apple in the olive oil until the onion is softened, about 4 minutes.

2. In a large saucepan over medium heat combine the apple and onion sauté with the vegetables, broth, and spices. Cover and simmer 20–25 minutes, or until the vegetables are tender.

3. Let cool a little, mix in the soy milk, and carefully blend in the blender in small batches. Serve warm.

Wild Greens Soup or Beverage

This recipe was created by Gayle Stolove, BS, RN, LMT, macrobiotic educator, personal chef, and founder of Wholly Macro, www.whollymacrobiotics.com.

INGREDIENTS | YIELDS 2–4 SERVINGS

1 cup kale, chopped

1 cup mustard greens, chopped

1 cup broccoli raab (rappini), chopped

1 cup watercress, chopped

1 cucumber, chopped

2 scallions, choppped

¼ cup grated carrot

1 tablespoon chopped cilantro

1½ cups spring water

¼ teaspoon sea salt

1. Heat water in a large pot to barely simmer, add greens (leave out the carrots, cucumber, and cilantro) for just 1 minute to barely cook. Drain them in a colander.

2. Then combine the greens with the cucumber, carrots, and cilantro and place into a blender. Blend until smooth. You can also make this soup raw and cool, which is a delicious beverage. Just place all the ingredients directly into blender.

Don't Be So Bitter!

In Eastern medicine wild greens with their natural bitterness stimulate the heart to contract. Kale and mustards have pronounced veins throughout their leaves, which are their own nutrient pathways. When you eat these greens you enhance your circulatory system as well, delivering fresh nutrients and oxygen throughout your body.

Cauliflower Creamy Soup

If using white beans instead of nuts, add a ½ piece ginger, minced, if desired. This recipe offers a suggested step of preroasting a garlic bulb which adds its own special flavors to your food.

INGREDIENTS | YIELDS 2–3 SERVINGS

1 bulb garlic for garlic roasting method, for sautéing option use 1–2 cloves chopped depending on garlic preferences.

1 teaspoon extra-virgin olive oil, and 2 additional teaspoons if roasting the garlic

½ onion, chopped

1 stalk celery

2 cups salt-free chicken or vegetable broth

½ cauliflower

½ cup cashews or walnuts, soaked in water to soften, or 1 cup cooked white beans mixed with ½ piece ginger, minced (optional)

⅓ cup soy milk

1 tablespoon chopped chives

1 tablespoon fresh parsley

¼ teaspoon paprika or pepper, or to taste

½ teaspoon sea salt

1. If using roasted garlic method, peel off the outer layers of skin from the garlic bulb, and cut off about ½ inch of the top of the bulb to expose the cloves; drizzle with 2 teaspoons of the olive oil, wrap in foil, and place in 400°F oven for 45 minutes. Peel and spoon out 1–3 cloves, depending on garlic preferences, to use for this recipe. Save the remaining roasted garlic, stored in the refrigerator, for another recipe, or as a great spread on pita bread, as a snack.

2. In a large stockpot combine the onions, roasted garlic, or peeled chopped 1 or 2 cloves raw garlic, and celery with 1 teaspoon olive oil and ¼ cup of the broth; cook to soften about 4–5 minutes.

3. Add the cauliflower, nuts or beans (and ginger, if using), and the rest of the broth; bring to boil, cover, and simmer for 15 minutes.

4. Let cool slightly. Add the soy milk. Blend in small batches in a blender with the herbs and spices.

Cocoa Loco Beverage

The chocolate flavor in this recipe will truly make you go loco for cocoa.

INGREDIENTS | YIELDS 1 SERVING

1 banana

½ cup soy milk

½ cup yogurt

1 tablespoon unsweetened cocoa powder

1 tablespoon honey, agave syrup, or stevia

1–2 pitted dried prunes or red dates

1 (2-ounce) scoop soy or whey protein powder

1 tablespoon ground flaxseed

1 cup water

2–3 ice cubes, to taste for desired "iciness"

Combine all the ingredients in a blender and blend until smooth. Pour into a glass and serve.

Fruit for Heart Health Beverage

This recipe lets you choose your favorite berry to include.
For a greener drink, add 1 cup of chopped kale or spinach.

INGREDIENTS | YIELDS 1 SERVING

1 cup fresh or frozen fruit (berries, cherries, melons, pears, grapes)

2 tablespoons soy or whey protein powder

½ cup yogurt or soy, rice, or nut milk

1 teaspoon ground flaxseed

1 tablespoon toasted wheat germ

1–2 dried pitted plums or red dates

1 cup water

2–3 ice cubes optional for desired level of "iciness"

Combine all the ingredients in a blender and blend until smooth. Pour into a glass and serve.

CHAPTER 10

Cleansing for Respiratory Problems

The pleasures of breathing . . . go beyond just allowing you to live. There is breathing in the smells of favorite foods cooking, breathing in the seasons outdoors with fireplaces smoking or chestnuts roasting, fall leaves dying, new spring growth, or summer flowers. And there is breathing well to enjoy games and exercise pastimes. And then there is easy breathing that relaxes you to fall peacefully asleep. What can spoil your life more—stop your play and activities— than a stuffy or runny nose that makes it hard to breathe? What can spoil a romantic moment quicker than labored breathing and wheezing?

Typical Breathing Issues

"Relax and take a deep breath"—words you may have heard from a yoga instructor or at a medical exam. Either way, its good advice. Oxygen is life's main nutrient. Someone once said, "The key to long life? Just don't stop breathing!" But breathing right, and deeply, isn't always as easy as it may sound.

FACT

In 1931 Otto Warburg was awarded the Nobel Prize for providing proof that many types of cancer cells are destroyed in a high-oxygen environment. The same is true of many germs, bacteria, and viruses. This is why it is important to keep the lungs healthy and to be able to breathe right.

The human body is made up of over 50 billion cells, all interacting with one another in biological processes and chemical reactions. And the force behind all of this is oxygen. If your breathing is not as full because of allergies, sinus problems, asthma, colds, flu, or any number of other respiratory issues, your cellular metabolism and the body's whole machinery will become slow and sluggish, and you will lose strength and vitality and feel the effects of aging more quickly.

Respiratory Infection

The Framingham Heart Study, a project of the National Heart, Lung, and Blood Institute and Boston University, reports that even under normal conditions, most people breathe at only 10 to 20 percent of what their optimal level could be. There are many conditions that affect normal breathing. One of the most common, and yet often preventable, is respiratory infection. Most people have at least one or two respiratory infections a year.

Respiratory infections can be as minor as a common cold, or as serious as bronchitis or pneumonia. Respiratory infections are usually divided into upper repository infections, which are the common infections of the nose, mouth, sinuses, and throat—the typical "coldlike" symptoms of which are stuffiness, runny nose, sore throat, cough, etc. Lower respiratory infections are a bit more serious and involve the lungs and bronchial tubes. Bronchitis and pneumonia are examples of lower respiratory infections. A diet high in the right nutrients and vitamins can boost the immune system and can lessen colds, flu, and respiratory infections; as well as improve lung function.

ESSENTIAL

Next time you a suffering from a stuffed up nose and head cold, you may wish to try a hot chili pepper. You know how that superhot jalapeño you had made your eyes water and nose run? It has that same effect when your sinuses are blocked due to colds, flu, or allergies. Capsaicin, the substance that gives chilies their hot bite, is also a natural decongestant, expectorant, and pain reliever.

Other Issues That Affect Respiratory Health

In addition to respiratory infections, other conditions that lead to difficulty breathing are asthma, allergies, and chronic obstructive pulmonary disease (COPD).

Asthma is a chronic disease of the respiratory system. It is the inflammation and narrowing of the bronchial tubes that carry air into the lungs. The inflammation can be severe in a so-called "asthma attack," leading to wheezing, difficulty breathing, tightness in the chest, and severe coughing. Asthma is very individualized, with attacks caused by many different things in different people, but it is almost always related to some type of allergy.

FACT

In a comparison study of people with asthma, those who had a diet low in whole grains and fish had episodes of wheezing almost 20 percent more than people whose diets were rich in these foods. Also, milk has been known to help ease the symptoms of asthma. It was often said it was because of the high amount of calcium; however, current research suggests it is actually the magnesium in milk that is the reason for its asthma-calming effect.

Allergies, particularly seasonal allergies such as hay fever, have the same symptoms of upper respiratory infections—sneezing, sore throats, sinus pressure, etc. But they are not caused by any kind of infection such as a virus or bacteria. Rather, the body launches an immune response to an allergen—such as pollen, dust, pet dander, or mold spores—similar to its reaction to an invading germ.

COPD is a progressive disease that causes difficulty with breathing, wheezing, and coughing. Cigarette smoking is the number one cause of COPD; yet, nonsmokers can develop the condition due to exposure to secondhand smoke and to other environmental toxins.

ALERT

Research has found that individuals with COPD can use up to 40 percent more energy per day than average folks because of their labored breathing. Being underweight could be as significant a health problem as being overweight. People who are underweight are at increased risk for infection and other health problems. Under certain circumstance, COPD patients have been encouraged to eat some high-calorie foods.

Improving your breathing can be key to improved health. Better "unblocked" breathing will increase your metabolism and all of your bodily functions. The more energizing oxygen you put into your body through better breathing, the more efficient your body will be at absorbing nutrients and creating revitalizing energy for your cells. Believe it or not, improved breathing can even help with weight loss, because when you continually breathe better you will need less food for energy and can comfortably go longer between meals!

Best Nutrients for Breathing

Worried about good health, no sick days, smelling nice aromas, having the breath to keep fit? Fortunately there are plenty of nutrients and good foods that can be added to your diet that will let you breathe easier!

Citrus fruits have long been known for their help in the prevention of respiratory issues such as colds and flu, and it turns out that it is not only because they are high in vitamin C. These fruits also contain compounds known as limonoids. Extracts made from limonoids found in citrus fruits have been found to protect lung tissue and reduce the mucus buildup typical of sufferers of COPD.

According to the American Lung Association, nearly 20 million Americans suffer from asthma. Studies have found that increasing consumption of whole grains and fish could reduce the risk of asthma by about 50 percent. However, researchers also point out that wheat can be a food allergen known to aggravate asthma, so other types of whole grains should be considered.

ESSENTIAL

Walnuts are one of the few nuts rich in omega-3s. If you are not a fish eater, consider sprinkling walnuts on salads or adding them to your cereal for an omega-3 breathing boost. Be aware of potential nut allergies, however.

It is the omega-3 fish oils that seem to be responsible for fish's calming effect on asthma. Omega-3s inhibit the production of cytokines, chemicals that are known to trigger airway restriction in asthmatics. On the other end of the spectrum are omega-6 oils, which actually stimulate the production of cytokines. According to the USDA the average American diet is very high in omega-6 oils; these are the oils used in most cookies, cakes, chips, and processed foods.

What Can Help

It may seem strange, but foods you eat really can affect your breathing, and the good news is research has shown that many common foods contain wonderful nutrients that work to improve lung and breathing abilities.

- The antioxidants found in many fruits and vegetables such as vitamins C, A, and E can minimize the severity of asthma attacks, can improve breathing, and reduce damage to bronchial tissues.

- Magnesium is an important nutrient that has been identified as calming the symptoms of asthma and improving lung function overall.
- Selenium, a mineral similar to magnesium in how it affects the body, also has been shown to have a positive effect on breathing, especially as related to the prevention of sinus and cold infections.
- Zinc has been shown to shorten how long colds last and their severity.
- Vitamin B_6 is essential to a healthy immune system. B_6 helps the body fight off all sorts of infections, and therefore may be helpful in boosting the body's resistance to colds, flu, and other respiratory infections.
- Folic acid, another B vitamin (B_9), also has been shown to help fight off respiratory infections. In fact, many believe it is the folic acid, and not the vitamin C, in orange juice that give it its cold-fighting ability.
- Quercetin, a powerful antioxidant found in onions, has been linked to the prevention of lung cancer. Fresh garlic also may prevent many respiratory ailments.
- Resveratrol and the other anti-inflammatory agents found in red wine that have been shown to lessen the risk of heart disease may help in preventing or lowering the risk of COPD.
- Carvacrol and thymol, two compounds found in thyme and oregano oil have been found to loosen phlegm in the lungs and relieve bronchial spasms.

ESSENTIAL

Thyme has long been used as a folk remedy for chest congestion and respiratory distress such as coughs and bronchitis. Recently, researchers pinpointed some of the compounds in thyme that are probably responsible for its healing effects. One of these is thymol. Thymol is also one of the key ingredients in that smelly and yet effective "vapor rub" smeared on the chest for colds in some home remedies.

What to Put in Your Shopping Cart

- **Vitamin A foods:** citrus fruit, tomatoes, carrots, mango, red bell pepper, spinach, collard greens, sweet potatoes, kale, turnip greens, collard greens, Swiss chard, milk, and eggs
- **Vitamin B$_6$ foods:** tuna, cod, salmon, snapper, halibut, chicken, liver, turkey, beef, banana, spinach, bell pepper, turnip greens, garlic, cauliflower, mustard greens, cremini mushrooms, Brussels sprouts, cabbage, asparagus, celery, kale, Swiss chard, and collard greens
- **Vitamin B$_9$ (folic acid) foods:** liver, lentils, pinto beans, garbanzo beans, black beans, navy beans, asparagus, spinach, collard greens, broccoli, beets, romaine, parsley, papaya, and string beans
- **Vitamin C foods:** bell peppers, parsley, broccoli, peppers, berries, citrus fruits, papaya, cauliflower, mustard greens, spinach, snow peas, cantaloupe, watermelon, tomatoes, zucchini, and celery
- **Limonoid foods:** oranges, grapefruits, and lemons, including white part and rind
- **Vitamin E foods:** mustard greens, Swiss chard, turnip greens, almonds, spinach, sunflower seeds, olives, papaya, and blueberries
- **Whole-grain foods:** barley, buckwheat, millet, rice, amaranth, kasha, quinoa, and lentils
- **Magnesium and folate foods:** beans, turmeric, spinach, squash, mustard greens, pumpkin, soybeans, sunflower seeds, flaxseeds, sesame seeds, green beans, cucumbers, celery, kale, black and navy beans, peppermint, and molasses
- **Selenium foods:** liver, Brazil nuts, snapper, cod, halibut, tuna, salmon, sardines, shrimp, barley, oats, mushrooms, sunflower seeds, eggs, turkey, lamb, and tofu
- **Omega-3 fatty acid foods:** salmon, flaxseed, walnuts, sardines, soybeans, halibut, snapper, scallops, shrimp, and tofu
- **Quercetin foods:** black and green tea, capers, apples, onion, red grapes, citrus fruit, grapefruit, peas, buckwheat, tomatoes, broccoli, leafy greens, and honey
- **Carvacrol and thymol foods:** oregano and thyme

How a Cleanse Can Help

Doing a cleanse for your respiratory system can help to maximize the way the lungs can get rid of impurities and help the whole body come work together to support the respiratory system.

Plan to do your cleanse for one to three days. Begin your day with 12–16 ounces of water with a squirt of lemon or lime juice and a teaspoon of ground flaxseed. Choose a breakfast, lunch, and dinner, and two snacks in between the meals. Later in this chapter are some suggested recipes. For your snacks, you could choose a blended drink of 1 celery, 1 cucumber, 1 cut-up orange, a small piece of fresh ginger, and water, or a few chunks of watermelon or other melon blended with water and ice. Use the white area of the watermelon as well and add a squeeze of lemon or lime juice. Make sure to drink your fluids every hour, including water and herbal teas.

Ginger tea can also be used to clear sinuses and treat any respiratory complaint. Holistic practitioners often recommend to be careful to not boil the fresh gingerroot for this tea, as its healing properties are diminished. Bring 4 cups of water to a boil in a saucepan. Peel a 2-inch piece of ginger and slice into thin strips. Once water is boiling, reduce to a very low simmer, then add the ginger and simmer for 20 minutes. Strain ginger from the liquid, and add honey and lemon to taste.

After the Cleanse

Following your cleanse, keep the following things in mind. Begin to increase your selection and amounts of solid foods. A great interim meal suggestion is made with cooked buckwheat kernels, or roasted kasha. You can make a fabulous pilaf with it by adding in any combinations of vegetables, fruits, nuts, or chicken. One variation is carrots, sweet potatoes or canned pumpkin, raisins, and nuts, finished off with Greek-style or soy yogurt.

Going forward, make sure you keep up your healthy behaviors:

- Keep your drinking/flushing habits alive with herbal teas and water.
- Do some exercise—both cardio and strength training. Aim for four times a week, and walk every day.

- A little percussion or light drumming on the rib cage can help to loosen up impurities in the lungs. You can do this lying down on your side, too.
- Breathing from your stomach rather than your chest is recommended as a better way to fill the lower parts of your lungs.
- Stretching is important. It increases oxygen and blood flow and decreases stress.

FACT

Family doctor, Dr. Harry Lechan, advises everyone at any age to daily expand the lungs by breathing in to the count of four, hold it, and let it out to the count of five. This fills up the tiny grape-like air sacks in the lungs and prevents them from shriveling and not inflating properly, allowing impurities to mount up and become like glue. Taking an extra count when breathing out helps to release all the impurities.

Remember that there are many, many wonderful and nutritious foods you can choose from that will help your lungs to be in the best of health, as well as the rest of your body. Using a wide variety of foods in your everyday diet is the way to make the most of what the earth has to offer you. By making the right food choices your lungs will thank you, and you'll breathe easier about your health and wellness.

Orange Pineapple Sunny Beverage

Some people are repulsed by juice with pulp in it, but that pulp has valuable nutrients in it that can assist in improving your respiratory system.

INGREDIENTS | YIELDS 1 SERVING

1 whole orange or 1 cup fresh-squeezed with pulp

1 cup chopped pineapple, papaya, or kiwi, or a mix

½ banana

1 cup water

1 teaspoon lemon juice

1 scoop whey protein powder, or ½ cup soaked and softened walnuts, almonds, or hazelnuts

2–3 ice cubes, if desired for "iciness"

Grated fresh ginger, cinnamon, or cayenne pepper, to taste (optional)

Combine all ingredients in a blender and blend until smooth. Pour into a glass and serve.

A Teatime Smooth Beverage

Green tea contains valuable nutrients and antioxidants that can help with all kinds of health issues. It's not caffeinated and leaves you feeling fresh, so consider swapping out your morning coffee for a cup of green tea.

INGREDIENTS | YIELDS 1 SERVING

1 cup of prepared green tea

1 cup water

1 banana

1 cup berries of your choice

1 (2-ounce) scoop protein powder or 2 tablespoons nut butter, or ¼ cup soaked, ground nuts

1–2 teaspoons ground flaxseed depending on desired need for regularity

½ cup chopped kale or spinach leaves

1–2 teaspoons honey, maple syrup, or stevia, or to taste

Combine all ingredients in a blender and blend until smooth. Pour into a glass and serve.

Carrot Apple Ginger Bisque

This recipe was created and recommended for cleansing of respiratory problems by Gayle Stolove, BS, RN, LMT, macrobiotic educator, personal chef, and founder of Wholly Macro, www.whollymacrobiotics.com.

INGREDIENTS | YIELDS 4–6 SERVINGS

4 cups spring water

1 cup rinsed red lentils

1 yellow onion, diced

6 carrots, diced

1 clove garlic, minced

3 Granny Smith apples, diced

2 tablespoons minced fresh ginger

¼ cup fresh lemon juice

Sea salt, to taste

1 tablespoon minced fresh parsley

1. Place water in pot and bring to boil.

2. Add the red lentils, onions, and carrots, and cook until soft, about 1 hour.

3. Turn off heat and add the remaining ingredients, except the parsley, to the pot.

4. Transfer the ingredients in batches to a blender or food processor and blend until smooth and creamy.

5. Garnish with minced parsley before serving.

Ginger Snap!

This bisque is delicious soup designed to cleanse the lungs and large intestine. This soup infuses the body with vitamin A via the carrots, which takes a great burden off the lungs and large intestine, while also utilizing the cleansing and healing qualities of fresh ginger and apples. Ginger also has natural antiseptic and antibacterial qualities, ensuring the health of the lungs and large intestine during this cleanse. As the ginger releases mucus and other toxins from the respiratory system, the fiber from the fresh apples and the red lentils comes along and sweeps everything through the large intestine and out of the body in perfect synchronicity.

Trusty True Chicken Wellness Soup

Chicken soup is not just for when you have the flu—this recipe is a great pick-me-up for lunch or dinner, and packs a nutrient punch to keep you breathing healthy. This soup freezes well, so save your extra servings for later.

INGREDIENTS | YIELDS 4–6 SERVINGS

1 (4-pound) chicken
7 cups cold water
1 package of chicken wings
1 large onion, chopped
1 sweet potato, chopped
2 parsnips, chopped
1 turnip, peeled and chopped
4 carrots, chopped
4 stalks celery, chopped
1 leek, chopped
1 bunch parsley
1 tablespoon chopped fresh dill
Sea salt and pepper, to taste

1. Clean the chicken well but leave on the skin. Put it in a large pot, cover with the water, and bring to a boil.

2. Add the rest of the ingredients, except the salt and pepper. Bring to a boil and simmer 3 hours. Using a strainer, skim off fat and impurities from the top.

3. Take out the chicken. The chicken is not used further for this soup, but you may save it for another use or add it in as a nutritious solid after your cleanse.

4. Cool a little, then blend the soup in a processor very carefully in small batches. Add salt and pepper to taste.

Achoo!

A Nebraska Medical Center researcher, Stephen Rennard, MD, has proven in a traditional clinical-style trial that chicken soup may help to prevent and does indeed lessen the severity of colds and flu. Soups the world over have long been used for their healing effect. Researchers believe, as in chicken soup, it is not any one ingredient that is responsible for the anti-inflammatory healing power of soup, but all the flavonoids and other nutrients that come from onions, carrots, garlic, oregano, chilies, tomatoes, and the other typical ingredients coming together.

Pea and Cress Soup

Which is better—fresh or frozen veggies? For this recipe, either fresh or frozen work just fine.

INGREDIENTS | YIELDS 3–4 SERVINGS

½ onion, diced

1–2 cloves garlic (depending on garlic preference), minced

1 tablespoon extra-virgin olive oil

1 bunch of watercress, washed and trimmed

2 cups fresh or frozen peas

1 small potato, peeled, diced small

4 cups vegetable stock

2 tablespoons chopped fresh mint

Salt and pepper, to taste

1. In a large pot over medium heat, sauté the onions and garlic in the olive oil until tender, about 4–5 minutes.

2. Add all the remaining ingredients, except the mint and salt and pepper, and bring to a boil; reduce heat and simmer 8–10 minutes.

3. Let cool a little and purée carefully in small batches, adding the mint. Add seasonings to taste. Pour into a serving bowl and enjoy.

Cool Cuke and Garden Beverage

Avocados are a great source of antioxidants, and their soft texture makes them easy to blend or mash. This recipe uses herbs and spices like cilantro and cumin to make the taste pop.

INGREDIENTS | YIELDS 1–2 SERVINGS

2 ripe avocados, diced and peeled

1 cucumber, seeded, peeled, and diced

1 tomato

¼ cup fresh lemon juice

2 sliced green onions

1 clove garlic, sliced

2 tablespoons cilantro

1 teaspoon ground cumin

1 cup water

1 cup vegetable stock

1 teaspoon ground flaxseed

Salt and pepper, to taste

Drizzle of extra-virgin olive oil, for garnish (optional)

1. Combine all ingredients in a blender and blend until smooth. Chill for 1 hour.

2. Serve with a drizzle of olive oil, if desired.

CHAPTER 11

Cleansing for Balanced Bacteria Levels

Friendly flora are tough and determined bacteria that want to "colonize" the gut and GI tract. This is a great thing because these friendly bacteria make and give your body vitamins K, B_{12}, and other vitamins, and stimulate development of some necessary GI tract tissues. They are the important "colonizers" you want to stake out claims in your GI tract, because they actually prevent "bad" bacteria, the bacteria that are pathogenic, from moving in by grabbing up space and nutrients. So, if there are more friendly flora colonizing, there will be less of the bad pathogens to take hold. The normal friendly flora have other ways to ward off bad bacteria as well, by making substances such as fatty acids and peroxides that can stop or kill the bad bacteria. And, the normal friendly flora stimulate the making of some natural antibodies—things that also prevent infection or invasion.

Typical Bacteria Issues

Germs and bacteria are often all lumped together as bad, as causes of disease and illness—which indeed, many of them are. But there is the normal flora bacteria that should be welcomed in, and not warded off, so these "good guys" can do their jobs in your body. The sad story is, many of today's lifestyle choices kill the good bacteria and/or disrupt the balance so that there are less friendly flora and more bad bacteria. Antibiotics, other medications, stress, food additives, overprocessed foods, lack of balanced nutrients in the diet—all contribute to disrupting the balance of friendly flora.

FACT

Our ancient Paleolithic ancestors seemed to know a lot more then we do about keeping the right "good bacteria/bad bacteria" balance. Recent archeological finds along the Texas-Mexico border reveal that prehistoric people ate more than 4½ pounds a day of prebiotic fiber.

Luckily, research has discovered some of the particular bacteria that are helpful, and they are part of the makeup of certain foods that you can make sure are included in your healthful diet.

Bacteria Hysteria

For a very long time modern medicine did not even understand germs and bacteria. People got sick, but the idea that something that couldn't even be seen was responsible for the sickness was too hard to believe. Even when microbes were discovered, and their link to infection known to be real, there were really no great treatments until the discovery of antibiotics in the late 1940s. This was a huge turning point for modern medicine. Until then, the best thing one could do about most bacterial infections was to eat well and live a healthy lifestyle to prevent them—and this worked well for people who were able to follow that plan. But, of course, not everyone is able to always follow that plan to the letter, and antibiotics became an easy way to get fast relief from bacterial infections. But things actually turned out a bit like science fiction. The widespread use of antibiotics has created more and more new bacteria that are drug resistant. So, drug companies have had to invent newer and more powerful drugs, and the more powerful the drugs, the more resistant the bugs become, and so on, and so on.

ALERT

Candida albicans is a bacteria that normally exists in the digestive system. In regular amounts it is not harmful; however, when it is allowed to grow, often due to overuse of antibiotics or a diet that throws off the good/bad bacteria balance, vaginal, mouth, or skin infections of candida can be the result.

In addition, more powerful drugs come with more side effects. And so, in the war against bacterial infections, it seems that the original ideas were the best where an "ounce of prevention" really *is* worth a "pound of cure." Many of the most common bacterial infections can be prevented or made less severe with the right diet and nutrition.

Good Bacteria and Bad Bacteria

People are bombarded by billions of bacteria every day. Some people are more susceptible than others. But the best way to prevent any bacterial infection from happening is to keep up a healthy immune system with proper nutrition and keeping the right good bacteria/bad bacteria balance. Not all bacteria are bad; in fact, some of the most common bacterial issues, vaginitis for example, can happen when the body's ratio of good to bad flora is off. This again is one of the problems with taking powerful antibiotics. These drugs can often kill off as much of the "good guys" as the bad guys when they are taken to fight infection.

FACT

So just how do "good bacteria" boost the immune system? Research suggests that it works almost like a natural vaccine. The body reacts to the presence of even good bacteria by making more B cells, which are the cells of the immune system that make antibodies to invading bacteria. It's as if the presence of good bacteria stimulates the immune system to gear up for battle.

Besides respiratory infections and urinary tract infections, some of the most common bacterial infections are:

- Vaginitis
- Candida
- Skin infections
- Strep infections

Problems with bacteria are also often caused by so-called food poisoning, such as E. coli and salmonella. But again, keeping that right balance between the good and bad bacteria in the digestive tract can help to prevent illness brought on by taking in any "bad" bacteria.

ESSENTIAL

In ancient times honey was used as an antibacterial ointment on wounds. Honey and bee pollen have been found to have an antibacterial effect, and are good ingredients to add to a nutritional battle against bad bacteria.

Bacteria are also the cause of body odors and bad breath that can also make surrounding people sick and uncomfortable. But fortunately the bacteria that cause these offending issues can also be helped with a healthy nutritional balance that ensures you have enough good bacteria and a healthy immune system.

Best Nutrients for Healthy Bacteria

Using nutritional methods to manage your daily exposure to bacteria and their potential harmful effects is like two sides of the same lucky coin. On one side, eating good foods can boost the levels of good bacteria that deal with the bad bacteria. On the other side, eating foods high in nutrients has been proven to boost the immune system. So if you can give your immune system the right boost and maintain the proper good/bad bacteria balance, your body will almost always be able to gain the upper hand over the bad bugs.

Vitamins

The powerful antioxidant nutrients vitamin E, vitamin B_{12}, vitamin C, vitamin A, beta-carotene, folic acid, and vitamin D and the minerals zinc, riboflavin, iron, copper, and selenium naturally boost the immune system. This helps your body ward off and deal with "bad" bacteria, by destroying free radicals and their damaging effects.

FACT

The fermentation process is caused by bacteria. You can thank friendly bacteria for treats such as sourdough bread, sour cream, and sauerkraut, which in German literally translates to "sour cabbage." But that pickled slaw is more than just good dressing for a hot dog; it also helps to promote healthy bacteria.

Glutamine, which is very helpful for muscle strength and in fighting fatigue, has also been shown to help the production of white blood cells. White blood cells are keys to the immune system.

Catechins, such as those found in green tea, are another dietary antioxidant that helps the immune system. When it comes to resisting bacteria, catechins generate the production of hydrogen peroxide, which is probably used in your home for its antibacterial properties.

Calling All Good Bacteria

Now for the other side of the coin—increasing your level of friendly bacteria. Probiotics are the live bacterial cultures found in yogurts. They are also found in buttermilk, certain kinds of cheeses, kefir, and sauerkraut. These foods have "good" bacteria that are normally found in the digestive system, on the skin, and in the vaginal and urinary tracts. They are there to ensure the proper working of these systems and to put a stop to "bad" bacteria. Eating probiotic-rich foods helps these good bacteria increase and leaves less room for the bad bacteria.

Prebiotics are found in foods that are not able to be totally digested. That may sound like a bad thing, but it is a good thing. Prebiotics can be found in insoluble fiber foods, and they "take up space" in the digestive track and do not let bad bacteria grow. They actually help the production of good bacteria, which are called *friendly flora*.

ALERT

Humans are a buffet for bacteria. There are bacteria that feast in the gut, the mouth, the feet, and skin. And all of these bacteria put out waste products, many of which can be smelly. Bacteria are responsible for most body odors. Rather than covering them up, you can minimize them by eating less sumptuous foods such as white bread and red meat.

Lactoferrin, a protein polypeptide found in milk and other dairy products, has been shown to be beneficial in maintaining a proper good/bad bacteria balance. In clinical studies lactoferrin seems to have an antibiotic effect and can inhibit the growth of various bad bacteria.

What to Put in Your Shopping Cart

Here are some foods that contain the best nutrients that will help you with your cleanse. Choose as many of them as you wish, and continue to choose them in your daily diet.

ANTIOXIDANTS:
- **Vitamin A foods:** citrus fruit, tomatoes, carrots, mango, red bell pepper, spinach, collard greens, sweet potatoes, kale, turnip greens, Swiss chard, milk, and eggs
- **Beta-carotene foods:** sweet potatoes, carrots, kale, spinach, turnip greens, winter squash, collard greens, cilantro, thyme, cantaloupe, romaine, and broccoli
- **Vitamin B_2 (riboflavin) foods:** liver, cremini mushrooms, yogurt, soybeans, spinach, milk, tempeh, eggs, romaine, and asparagus
- **Vitamin B_9 (folic acid) foods:** liver, lentils, pinto beans, garbanzo beans, black beans, navy beans, asparagus, spinach, collard greens, broccoli, beets, romaine, parsley, papaya, and string beans

- **Vitamin C foods:** citrus fruits, strawberry, lemon, papaya, grapefruit, cantaloupe, raspberry, watermelon, pineapple, parley, broccoli, bell peppers, cauliflower, mustard greens, kiwi, snow peas, and zucchini
- **Vitamin D foods:** salmon, sardines, shrimp, milk, cod, and eggs
- **Vitamin E foods:** mustard greens, Swiss chard, spinach, olives, turnip greens, sunflower seeds, almonds, papaya, blueberries, and wheat germ

MINERALS:

- **Iron foods:** Swiss chard, spinach, thyme, turmeric, romaine, molasses, tofu, dill, parsley, basil, green beans, and wheat germ
- **Copper foods:** liver, cremini mushrooms, molasses, Swiss chard, spinach, sesame seeds, turnip greens, mustard greens, kale, and summer squash
- **Zinc foods:** liver, sea vegetables, pumpkin seeds, spinach, yeast, lamb, beef, summer squash, asparagus, Swiss chard, wheat germ, and brewer's yeast
- **Selenium foods:** liver, Brazil nuts, snapper, cod, halibut, tuna, salmon, sardines, shrimp, barley, oats, mushrooms, sunflower seeds, eggs, turkey, lamb, tofu, and wheat germ
- **Glutamine foods:** beef, chicken, fish, beans, and dairy
- **Catechins:** green tea, red grapes, and red wine
- **Lactoferrin:** low fat and fat free milk, whey products
- **Fiber foods:** fresh fruits, especially pears and apples, fresh vegetables, all whole grains, nuts, bran, flaxseeds, and wheat germ
- **Whole grains:** brown rice, buckwheat, corn, millet, quinoa, whole wheat, oats, and barley
- **Healthy fats including omega-3s:** olive oil, flaxseed oil, flaxseeds, salmon, walnuts, sardines, halibut, snapper, soybeans, and tofu
- **Probiotics and prebiotics:** yogurt, kefir, kimchi, tempeh, bananas, chicory root, onions, leeks, fruit, soybeans, sweet potatoes, and asparagus

How a Cleanse Can Help

Of course, as a living being everything about you is alive—and that includes bacteria. Nothing to be afraid of, because billions of them have always been and need to be on your skin, in your mouth, respiratory tract, and gut—from head to toe you are loaded with bacteria. And like the saying goes, you get the good with the bad. There are different kinds of bacteria on the skin, keeping the skin healthy by taking up residence and space so that dangerous pathogens don't get hold. Sometimes bacteria can cause issues such as warts or athlete's foot. Other bacteria make use of sweat to make body odors. Others keep genitalia healthy by warding off candida and other infections.

ALERT

A noticeable shift in the good/bad bacteria balance of the gut could be a possible indicator of future colon cancer, according to a study published by the University of North Carolina at Chapel Hill School of Medicine. The researchers found that when the balance tips in favor of the "bad" bacteria, those bacteria make toxic waste in the colon that could lead to cancer.

Hopefully, there's a nice balance always going on so that the good ones are keeping the bad ones out and in check. But changes in this balance can be responsible for a host of issues. Changes in balance can be the result of taking antibiotics, other medications, food additives, stress, and many things that happen in the typical American life. So, it is a wise thing to take the time to leave things behind that may upset your necessary balance and put into your body some healthy nutrients that all contribute to keeping pathogens in check.

Plan to do your cleanse from one to three days. Begin your day with 12–16 ounces of water with a squirt of lemon or lime juice and 1 teaspoon of ground flaxseed. Choose a breakfast, lunch, and dinner, and two in-between snacks/light meals. Some recipes are suggested later in this chapter.

For your in-betweeners, you could also choose a blended drink of 1 celery, 1 cucumber, 1 cut-up orange, a small piece of fresh ginger, and water, or a few chunks of watermelon or other melon, or a handful of strawberries blended with water and ice. If using watermelon, do use the white area of the watermelon as well and add a squeeze of lemon or lime juice. Or, you could blend up a dollop of fat-free plain yogurt with cucumber and fresh dill, with water and ice.

ESSENTIAL

Gingerols are volatile oils in the gingerroot. Ginger has long been known to soothe stomach distress, and it is now believed that the gingerols may be responsible for destroying bad bacteria in the gut and helping more good bacteria to take hold.

Another beverage suggestion is a hot cocoa made with water, 1 tablespoon of unsweetened cocoa, ¼ cup soy or fat-free milk, and stevia to sweeten if desired. Make sure to drink your fluids every hour, or ½ hour, including water and herbal teas.

After the Cleanse

Following your cleanse, here are some things to keep in mind:

- **Begin to increase your selection and amounts of solid foods.** A great interim meal suggestion is to spread a slice of whole-grain pita (or rice crackers for wheat allergies) with 1 teaspoon of hummus, and top with a ½ can of mashed sardines in olive oil or tomato sauce and a slice of tomato. Or, another meal suggestion is made with cooked buckwheat kernels, or roasted kasha. You can make a fabulous pilaf with it by adding in any combinations of vegetables, fruits, nuts, or chicken. One variation is carrots, sweet potato or canned pumpkin, raisins, and nuts, finished off with Greek-style or soy yogurt (if allergy permits).
- **Always make sure your system has important probiotics and prebiotics.** Dairy sources include yogurt, kefir, and cottage cheese. Nondairy sources include tofu, soy yogurt, miso, tempeh, and sauerkraut.
- **Fiber is crucial in any healthy diet.** Fruits, vegetables, nuts, and whole grains are excellent sources.
- **Keep your drinking/flushing habits alive with herbal teas and water.**

- **Do some exercise—both cardio and strength training.** Aim for four times a week, and walk every day.
- **Stretching is important.** It increases oxygen and blood flow, and decreases stress.

ALERT

Some types of bacteria are the number one cause of bad breath. Keep your mouth as unfriendly an environment to bacteria growth as you can by brushing and flossing often to remove food trapped between the teeth, and rinse well.

Remember that there are many, many wonderful and nutritious foods you can choose from that will help your bacteria balance to be in the best of health, as well as the rest of your body. Using a wide variety of foods in your everyday diet is the way to make the most of what the earth has to offer.

Your body will thank you for making the right food choices, by becoming a nice, welcome home to friendly bacteria, and a place the bad germs want to avoid!

Breakfast with Appeal

Fruit peels, like apple and orange peels, are chock-full of fiber and a great source of nutrients, so think twice before you peel and toss.

INGREDIENTS | YIELDS 1 SERVING

1 banana

1 apple or pear, cored and chopped

1 tablespoon sesame tahini

½ cup soy, rice, or almond milk

¼ cup tofu

1–2 teaspoons ground flaxseed depending on your needs for regularity

2 tablespoons toasted wheat germ

1 cup water

2–3 ice cubes (optional) for desired level of "iciness"

1–2 teaspoons stevia (optional)

1–2 teaspoons crumbled dried orange peel (optional)

Combine all ingredients in a blender. Blend until smooth. Pour into a glass and serve.

Holiday Breakfast Anytime

*The taste of nutmeg not only reminds you of the holidays,
but gets your body moving and grooving to wash out bad bacteria.*

INGREDIENTS | YIELDS 1 SERVING

½ cup pineapple (fresh or unsweetened canned)

1 carrot

1–2 dried, pitted prunes

¼ cup raw cashews, soaked in water to soften

1 teaspoon grated ginger

⅓ cup mashed baked sweet potato

2 teaspoons ground flaxseed

½ cup fat-free milk

1 cup soy, rice, or almond milk

¼ teaspoon cinnamon, if desired

¼ teaspoon curry, if desired

⅛ teaspoon nutmeg, if desired

1 cup water, and 2–3 ice cubes if "iciness" is desired

Place all ingredients in a blender. Blend until smooth. Pour into a glass and serve.

Okra Okay Soup

Okra is not only high on the nutrient list, it gives a dish a wonderful creaminess.

INGREDIENTS | YIELDS APPROXIMATELY 3–4 SERVINGS

2 pitted dried prunes or dried apricots

2 cups water

½ cup chopped celery

2 cups frozen cut okra

2 cups chopped spinach or chard

1 cup chopped onion

½ cup soy milk

¼ cup brown or wild rice

¼ cup raisins

1 teaspoon lemon juice

1. Soak dried fruit in the water overnight. Combine the fruit and the soaking water with all the other ingredients in a covered pot and simmer until the rice is mushy, about 1 hour. Let cool slightly.

2. Add to a blender in batches and blend carefully until smooth. Serve in bowls.

Reddy Cold Soup

This sweet and savory soup covers a range of great nutrients to perk you up.

INGREDIENTS | YIELDS 1 SERVING

½ cucumber
½ red bell pepper
¼ cup chopped onion, any type
½ cup chopped fresh basil
½ clove garlic, minced
1 teaspoon lemon juice
1 orange, sliced into sections
1 vine-ripened tomato
2 teaspoons extra-virgin olive oil
1 cup water
¼ cup tofu
¼ cup ground sunflower seeds

Place all ingredients in a blender. Blend until smooth. Serve in bowls.

Beans and Vegetable Soup

This filling soup is packed with the good nutrients of legumes.

INGREDIENTS | YIELDS 3–4 SERVINGS

½ cup dried kidney or navy beans, rinsed, or 1 cup canned beans, drained and rinsed

3 cups vegetable broth or water

1 large tomato

1 stalk celery, chopped small

1 carrot, chopped small

1 clove garlic, minced

½ onion (white, yellow, or red), chopped small

2 tablespoons tomato paste

1 tablespoon extra-virgin olive oil

1½ cups frozen cut okra

1 teaspoon thyme

1 teaspoon oregano

1 teaspoon cumin

Salt and pepper, to taste

¼ cup nonfat, plain Greek-style yogurt

1 teaspoon lime juice

1. If using dry beans, place the beans in the broth or water in a large pot and bring to a boil for 2 minutes. Then cover and let stand for 1 hour.

2. Add the vegetables and seasonings to the beans and water. If using dry beans, simmer 1 hour, or until the beans are soft. If using canned beans, simmer 10–15 minutes.

3. Cool slightly and blend carefully in batches. Serve with yogurt and lime juice swirled in.

CHAPTER 12

Cleansing for Head Pain and Congestion

Sometimes that terrible construction zone with the jackhammers buzzing and anvils clanging steel bars together is all happening inside your head. Your head sits on top of your shoulders, but there are times when it feels like it contains all of the above—weighing it down so much you can't even hold it up. And even lying down doesn't help to quiet the mayhem inside your head.

Typical Head Issues

You might already know the certain circumstances that can give you a pain in the head, but there are probably more that you wish you knew about. Foresight helps not to have as many regrets in the head pain and congestion department, and there is evidence culled from health professionals that offer plans for nutrients you can put into your diet, or take out, that can also help.

ESSENTIAL

Why people get headaches is a very individual thing. This is especially true of headaches caused by food allergies or sensitivities. Medical practitioners and head pain specialists recommend keeping a "headache diary" to see what is being eaten and drunk during flare-ups to help figure out what foods might be your triggers.

There is a real path you can follow for your own special head. No two heads are alike. Head pain nutrients are chosen by you to twist that nozzle of "triggers" away from your head. Trying to keep up with all of the latest information about diet, nutrition, and wellness can sometimes seem like a real headache—but the truth is, head pain can be very much related to the foods that you are and are not eating.

Types of Headaches

There is really no single kind or type of "headache." A headache can build slowly, or it can come on suddenly with all the fury of thunder. Medicine identifies headaches as basically belonging to one of three main head pain syndromes: tension headache, cluster headache, and migraine. But no matter what you call it, or its source, a headache can easily get in the way of your daily activities. Severe and recurring headaches can be very debilitating. Headaches often coexist with some other uncomfortable symptoms. With migraines, for example, there may also be nausea and more sensitivity to light and sound during an attack.

When there is head pain, the first thing many people do is reach for the bottle of some over-the-counter (OTC) pain reliever. Overuse them, even aspirin, and you will encounter a number of negative side effects. Acetaminophen (Tylenol) and Ibuprofen (Motrin/Advil) have been linked to kidney and liver problems. Besides their possible side effects, such pain relievers treat only the symptom—head pain—and do nothing to get at the root cause of the headache. Many of the worst head pain issues can be lessened or eliminated by understanding what causes headaches and making lifestyle and diet adjustments.

ESSENTIAL

Many headaches are caused by dehydration. Few people drink enough water, and walk around mildly dehydrated, which accounts for headaches, weakness, and a variety of other problems. Besides upping water intake, eat more foods rich in water, such as watermelons and cucumbers. This way you are not only taking in water to fight dehydration headaches, but also vitamins and minerals such as magnesium that are known to relieve head pain.

Tension Headaches

Tension headaches are probably the most common type—those occasional headaches that everyone suffers from time to time. A tension headache is basically pain in the head, scalp, or neck. The pain of a tension headache is usually not on just one side of the head, but kind of hurts all over. The feeling of a tension headache is usually described as tightness. Tension headaches tend to start slowly and build in strength over time. Tension headaches that happen more than two or three times a week are said to be chronic. Often chronic tension headaches can be caused by too much medication for the headaches, and the person gets what are called *rebound headaches*, after the pain relievers have worn off. Rebound is another reason why treating headaches, especially ongoing headaches, with OTC medications may not be the best thing to do. Tension headaches come from feeling physically and/or mentally tense. Physical tension that causes headaches is usually from tensed muscles in the neck or shoulders. Emotional tension such as stress, depression, and anxiety can all lead to tension headaches. Certain foods can also trigger tension headaches.

Cluster Headaches and Migraines

More severe than tension headaches are cluster headaches. Cluster headaches are mainly on one side of the head. Eye tearing or blood spots in the eye on the same side as the pain often accompanies cluster headaches, as does a runny nose. It is unclear what causes cluster headaches, but current research suggests it has to with the body producing a histamine reaction, such as in allergies. Cluster headaches usually come on very quickly and are also usually very painful. Most research estimates that cluster headaches are from the body reacting to something, or lack of something, such as a particular nutrient. Recommendations are often made to keep a "headache journal" for people who get cluster headaches to try to find out their particular triggers.

ALERT

If you get headaches from drinking red wine and think that switching to a "sulfite free" variety will solve your problem, it may not. Wine and medical experts agree that those who experience migraine or headaches after drinking red wine are more likely to be reacting to a chemical in the wine called *tyramine*. Tyramine is still present in sulfite-free wines. It can also be found in aged cheeses, chocolate, sour cream, pickled foods, and sauerkraut.

Often the most incapacitating type of headache is the migraine. Like a cluster headache, migraines are usually on one side of the head. There are usually not eye or nose issues with migraines, but often nausea, vomiting, and sensitivity to light are part of a migraine. Migraine sufferers also report seeing an "aura," or an unusual flash of light, just before a migraine begins. Migraines are very common, with 11–12 out of every 100 people suffering from them. Migraines affect more women than men and are caused by a change in brain activity. Things that seem to trigger the change in brain activity that leads to migraine can be certain foods, stress, or emotional distress. Most recent medical information on migraines indicate that the problem begins in the brain itself, with a shift in the levels of certain brain chemicals, and this shift causes a constriction of blood vessels.

Best Nutrients to Reduce or Eliminate Head Pain

Headaches are kind of like snowflakes—no two are alike. But that is where the similarity ends. Where snowflakes are soft, and gentle, and refreshing, headaches are brutal, thunderous, and painful. Most people turn to the medicine cabinet and the bottle of Tylenol, ibuprofen, or aspirin for relief. But what if there was a better way to prevent the pain before it starts? There is. A number of vitamins, minerals, and other nutrients have been found that can help prevent headaches. Adding more of them to your daily diet may help your problems with head pain.

Vitamin B

B vitamins are among the most essential of nutrients to head pain sufferers. In general, all of the vitamin Bs have been proven to help the body deal better with stress—a major cause of tension headaches.

Specifically, vitamin B_1, also known as thiamin, is great for headache sufferers of all types. B_1 boosts the production of cellular energy, and it seems to have a calming effect on migraines and allergy or histamine related headaches such as cluster headaches.

FACT

The amino acid tryptophan helps the body to produce vitamin B_3, and it also keeps up serotonin levels. Because of its important role for serotonin levels, tryptophan deficiency has been linked to poor sleep patterns, anxiety, depression, and migraine headaches. An excellent food source of tryptophan is brown rice. Others include soy protein, cottage cheese, turkey, and peanuts.

Niacin, or vitamin B_3, has been shown to open blood vessels, so it is a good way to prevent headaches, such as tension headaches and some types of cluster and migraine headaches that are caused by restricted blood flow. Vitamins B_5 and B_6 strengthen the adrenal gland and stabilize hormone production and the production of neurotransmitters such as serotonin. New research has shown that migraine and cluster headaches are related to hormonal and neurotransmitter imbalances. Vitamins B_5 and B_6 can help to ward off these types of headaches.

Vitamin C

Vitamins C and E, both powerful antioxidants, can help with head pain that is the result of oxidative stress. This is particularly true of headaches brought on by food allergies or sensitivities, as it is the free radicals in these foods that often are responsible for the head pain. In addition to its antioxidative effect, vitamin E also enhances blood flow, and therefore can help to prevent tension headaches.

Electrolytes

Keeping up a good level of electrolytes such as potassium and magnesium in the blood also seems to keep away certain kinds of headaches. Magnesium in particular has been found to help prevent or minimize migraine pain. One reason science has given for the experience of head pain is "overactive nerves." This is partially responsible for migraines, as well as that feeling of "raw nerves," or nervous tension. What these conditions are describing is the invasion of calcium into nerve cells, which causes them to overactivate, or "fire" more than normal. And then this causes muscles and blood vessels to constrict, leading to head pain. Magnesium has been found to help to control headaches because it is a natural "calcium blocker." In the body, magnesium binds to calcium and helps to take it from the blood, so it calms those "raw nerves."

Proteins and Omega-3s

In addition to these vital nutrients, a proper balanced diet is critical to prevent headaches. Lack of protein especially in the morning has been identified as a cause of many headaches. Eating too many fried foods and processed foods has many health ramifications, not the least of which is headaches. Omega-3 fatty acids, such as those found in fish, have been shown to help with some types of head pain. Natural "folk remedies" for head pain that have been shown to be as effective as over-the-counter pain medications include, lemon juice, ginger, and cinnamon. The natural anti-inflammatory bromelain, found in pineapples, has been shown to be as effective as nonsteroidal anti-inflammatory drugs (NSAIDS) for various forms of pain, including head pain.

What to Put in Your Shopping Basket

Here are some of the best nutrient-rich foods that can help you with your cleanse. Choose many of these for your cleanse, and continue to keep on selecting these foods for use in your daily diet.

- **Foods with vitamin B_1 (thiamin):** asparagus, romaine, mushrooms, spinach, sunflower seeds, celery, tuna, green peas, tomato, eggplant, Brussels sprouts, celery, and watermelon
- **Foods with vitamin B_2 (riboflavin):** liver, cremini mushrooms, yogurt, beef, soybeans, spinach, milk, tempeh, eggs, romaine, and asparagus
- **Foods with vitamin B_3 (niacin):** chicken, tuna, salmon, mushrooms, liver, halibut, lamb, turkey, cremini mushrooms, sardines, and asparagus
- **Foods with vitamin B_5:** liver, cauliflower, mushrooms, sunflower seeds, cremini mushrooms, yogurt, corn, broccoli, squash, and eggs
- **Foods with vitamin B_6:** tuna, cod, salmon, snapper, halibut, chicken, liver, turkey, beef, banana, spinach, bell peppers, turnip greens, garlic, cauliflower, mustard greens, cremini mushrooms, Brussels sprouts, cabbage, asparagus, celery, kale, Swiss chard, and collard greens
- **Foods with vitamin B_9 (folic acid):** liver, lentils, pinto beans, garbanzo beans, black beans, navy beans, asparagus, spinach, collard greens, broccoli, beets, romaine, parsley, papaya, and string beans
- **Foods with vitamin C:** bell peppers, parsley, broccoli, peppers, berries, citrus fruits, papaya, strawberries, cauliflower, mustard greens, spinach, snow peas, cantaloupe, watermelon, tomato, zucchini, and celery
- **Foods with vitamin E:** mustard greens, Swiss chard, turnip greens, almonds, spinach, sunflower seeds, olives, papaya, and blueberries
- **Foods with magnesium:** beans, turmeric, spinach, squash, and mustard greens
- **Foods with tryptophan:** wheat germ, cottage cheese, eggs, duck, turkey, granola, chicken, black-eyed peas, walnuts, almonds, sesame

seeds, Swiss and Gruyère cheese, shrimp, tamari, cremini mushrooms, cod, tuna, snapper, halibut, mustard greens, spinach, tofu, banana, beef liver, sardines, salmon, soybeans, mustard seeds, cauliflower, black beans, kidney beans, and milk

- **Foods with omega-3 fatty acids:** salmon, flaxseed, walnuts, sardines, soybeans, halibut, tofu, and snapper
- **Herbal teas:** peppermint and ginger

How a Cleanse Can Help

The same way head pain can mount and intensify with a stronger and stronger pounding, so too can the free radicals, allergens, and other substances that can cause head pain buildup in your body over time. By doing a cleanse, you can put yourself on a path that starts to get your head to say "ahhhh."

Begin your day with a large glass of water with a squirt of lemon or lime juice. Choose a breakfast, lunch, and dinner. Some recipes are suggested later in this chapter. Choose two snacks in between meals. A snack suggestion for anytime is a blend of 1 or 2 ounces of watermelon, cantaloupe, or cucumber and water, or add ¼ cup yogurt and/or ¼ cup nuts or seeds soaked in water to soften. Or, you could always use the plain vegetable broth you make yourself. Be sure to drink eight to ten glasses of fluids a day using teas and water. Don't let yourself feel hungry, because that will only add to your headaches. Aim to do your cleanse for one to three days.

After the Cleanse

Following your cleanse, here are some things to keep in mind:

- **Begin to increase your selection and amounts of solid foods.** A great interim meal is chickpeas or garbanzo beans, cooked with mushrooms, curry spices, and chopped walnuts, combined with brown rice. Or, spread a slice of whole-grain pita (or rice crackers) with 1 teaspoon of hummus, and top with a ½ can of mashed sardines or ¼ cup mashed canned salmon or tuna, and a tomato slice. Or, another meal choice is made with cooked buckwheat kernels, or roasted kasha. You can make a fabulous pilaf with it by adding in any combinations of vegetables, fruits, nuts, or chicken. One variation is carrots, sweet potato or canned pumpkin, dried apricots, and nuts, finished off with Greek-style or soy yogurt.

- **Your system likes important probiotics and prebiotics.** Dairy sources include yogurt, kefir, and cottage cheese. Nondairy sources include tofu, soy yogurt, miso, tempeh, and sauerkraut.
- **Keep your drinking/flushing habits alive with herbal teas and water.**
- **Do some exercise—both cardio and strength training.** Aim for four times a week, and walk every day. Mild exercise such as a brisk walk, even during a headache experience, can help because it releases the body's endorphins, which are natural painkillers.
- **Stretching is important.** It increases oxygen and blood flow, and decreases stress.
- **Eating regularly is important, and breakfast is really the most helpful.** Eating a good protein for breakfast can help ward off headaches as you continue through the day.
- **Massage is often helpful.** Headache sufferers often find it hard to believe, but a foot massage can be helpful in relieving pain.

Quinoa Queen for Breakfast and Anytime

Not enough protein has been noted as one cause of some common headaches. Quinoa is a good source of protein, especially for vegans. Quinoa has an added bonus for migraine headache sufferers: it is high in magnesium, a mineral that has been shown to relax blood vessels.

INGREDIENTS | YIELDS 1 SERVING

¼ cup quinoa

½ cup water

¼ cup rolled oats

1 cup berries (strawberries, blueberries, raspberries)

⅓ cup ground almonds, walnuts, or cashews

2 teaspoons honey

1 cup milk of your choice

1 teaspoon ground flaxseed

2–3 ice cubes, if desired for "iciness"

1. First, prepare the quinoa by rinsing it well with water.

2. Then put in pan with the ¼ cup water; bring to a boil, cover, and simmer 15 minutes (or follow package directions).

3. Let the quinoa cool. Add it along with all the other ingredients to blender and blend until smooth. Pour into a glass and serve. Can be a warm or a cold beverage.

Cottage Pleasure Beverage

Honey is a great way to sweeten your food without adding refined sugar or artificial sweetener. You can also use watermelon, melon, or cucumbers in place of the berries in this recipe.

INGREDIENTS | YIELDS 1 SERVING

1 cup berries of your choice
½ cup fat-free cottage cheese
Drizzle of honey
1 cup romaine or kale
1 cup water
2 tablespoons rolled oats
1 teaspoon ground flaxseed
2–3 Ice cubes, if desired for "iciness"

Place all ingredients in a blender. Blend until smooth. Pour into a glass and serve.

Cauliflower Cookin' Good Soup

Curcumin, the active ingredient in turmeric, has been found to have a similar anti-inflammatory effect to aspirin, and has been used to treat headaches in the Ayurvedic (traditional Indian medicine) tradition.

INGREDIENTS | YIELDS 3 SERVINGS

1 large leek, white and tender green part only, sliced thin

2 teaspoons extra-virgin olive oil

1 small baking potato, peeled and chopped coarse

1 teaspoon curry

3 cups cauliflower florets

½ cup mushrooms

½ cup chopped celery

1½ cups broth or water

Sea salt and pepper, to taste

½ cup plain, nonfat Greek-style or soy yogurt

1. In a large pot over moderately low heat, cook the leeks in the olive oil, stirring until partially wilted, about 7 minutes.

2. Add the chopped potato and curry; stir and cook another 3 minutes.

3. Add the cauliflower, mushrooms, celery, and broth or water. Bring to a boil, cover, and simmer until the vegetables are very soft, about 30 minutes.

4. Let cool a little; purée in a blender carefully in batches. Season to taste with salt and pepper. Swirl in 1 tablespoon yogurt when serving.

A Pear of Good Foods Beverage

Pears are very low on the glycemic chart, so they do not spike the blood sugar,
yet they add delicious sweetness.

INGREDIENTS | YIELDS 1 SERVING

1 pear

½ cucumber

½ avocado

1 teaspoon fresh mint leaves

1 stalk celery, remove strings

1 green onion

1 teaspoon lemon juice

1 cup water

2–3 ice cubes, if desired for "iciness"

Combine all the ingredients in a blender and blend until smooth. Pour into a glass and serve.

Veggie Broth

Making your own broth will save your head the possible pains of commercial varieties that have potentially unfriendly additives.

INGREDIENTS | YIELDS 5 CUPS

2–3 tablespoons extra-virgin olive oil

1 cup chopped green onions

1 cup chopped carrots

1 cup chopped celery

2 quarts water

1–2 cloves of garlic, depending on your garlic preference

5 peppercorns

1 cup chopped parsnip

1 cup chopped sweet potato or white potato

1 cup chopped zucchini

1 cup chopped mushrooms

1 cup chopped green or red bell pepper

1. Heat the oil in a large stockpot and add the green onions, carrots, and celery. Saute over medium heat for 4–5 minutes.

2. Add the water, the rest of the vegetables and herbs and bring to a boil, then simmer for 1 hour.

3. Carefully strain the vegetables out and discard, and your broth is left behind. You can also pour some broth into ice-cube trays and freeze for adding to other recipes.

4. Keep the broth refrigerated for 1 week, or 2 months in the freezer. You can use it as a delicious and nutritious base for cooking your rice and other grains, and bean and vegetable soups. Use it to prepare the Lemony Egg Soup later in this chapter.

Lemony Egg Soup

This soup feels light on the tongue, but has great nutritional weight with excellent protein, B vitamins, and tryptophan in the egg alone!

INGREDIENTS | YIELDS 1 SERVING

1 cup Veggie Broth (Chapter 12)
1 egg
1 teaspoon fresh lemon juice

1. Heat broth in a saucepan to boiling.

2. Beat together the egg and lemon juice. Beat in a little of the hot broth into the egg and then add to the rest of the broth.

Mushroom Pumpkin Cashew Soup

You don't have to wait until Halloween or Thanksgiving to enjoy the nutrient-rich goodness of pumpkin.

INGREDIENTS | YIELDS 3–4 SERVINGS

1 tablespoon extra-virgin olive oil

1 cup thinly sliced mushrooms

½ cup chopped green onions

2½ cups broth

1 (16-ounce) can pumpkin purée (or use 1 cooked butternut squash, chopped)

¾ cup frozen orange juice concentrate, thawed

1 cup raw cashews blended with 1 cup water to "cream," or 1 cup soy or fat-free milk

Cinnamon, to taste

Sea salt and pepper, to taste

1. Place the olive oil in skillet over medium heat. Add the mushrooms and green onions, and cook until tender, about 3–4 minutes.

2. Add the broth, pumpkin puree or squash, orange juice concentrate, cashew cream (or milk), and seasonings.

3. Simmer (do not boil) 10 minutes.

4. Cool a little. Add all to blender carefully in batches and blend until smooth.

CHAPTER 13

Cleansing for Better Focus and Concentration

Even after a good night's sleep many people wind up sleep-walking through the day with a feeling of being dazed and confused that can leave you unfulfilled. It starts with that thick-headed foggy feeling, and then as the morning goes on, you're listening to somebody or something and you are in the embarrassing situation of realizing that you just weren't able to pay attention well enough to know what was going on. Embarrassing situations like this can happen: your boss is explaining the quarterly reports, or your best friend is describing a unique experience, your mom is asking you for advice . . . and all of a sudden you realize they finished speaking and all you think of is "what?"

Typical Concentration Issues

There's more to focusing and concentrating than being able to look wide-eyed at a speaker or a document. There's more to remembering than trying to use rhymes or having special places to put things. These are tricks that are supposed to help with focus and concentration, but there are better ways with no tricks involved to give your brain the good tools it needs to focus and concentrate. Study after study has given honest evidence of nutrients that really work to improve the precious brain cells and get signals to the brain easier and faster.

Memory Loss

It happens to everyone. You walk into a room and forgot what you went in for. You press a cell phone number, and while it's connecting you actually forget who you called, until you recognize the voice on the other end. And what about those car keys that just seem to keep getting up and walking away from wherever it was you put them down! Such momentary memory lapses or cognitive difficulties are very common, and they don't just happen to the elderly. Memory loss and difficulty thinking or concentrating can be more related to what's on your dinner table than your age, and in fact you can give yourself a good nutritional "brain boost" at any age.

FACT

One of the sources of the cognitive problems in Alzheimer's patients is a buildup of chemicals called *homocysteines* in their brains. Homocysteines are destroyed by vitamins B_6 and B_{12} and folate, all of which are found in green superfoods such as broccoli.

Long-term or severe memory loss and cognitive difficulties can be symptoms of a serious medical condition, especially if there is also head pain, dizziness, blurred vision, or other symptoms. Anyone experiencing such symptoms should seek professional medical attention immediately. However, mild problems or difficulty from time to time with concentration and memory are almost always the result of stress, diet, and lifestyle.

Attention Sappers

In addition to memory loss, one of the other most commonly described mild cognitive difficulties is the ability to concentrate. There are many reasons why adults today have more trouble than ever concentrating. One big reason, of course, is the typical "multitasking" lifestyle of juggling work, home, family, and other personal obligations.

ALERT

When looking for that nutritional brain boost, don't overlook water. Proper hydration is as necessary to clear thinking, memory, and cognitions as proteins and amino acids. The brain is 85 percent water. Even a little dehydration can cause the transmission of electrical impulses in the brain to lessen.

What exactly is concentration? It is the brain's ability to focus on a task at hand without being distracted by other things. When you are at a "peak performance" level of concentration on whatever task, that task takes less time, is easier, is completed with fewer mistakes, and is easier the next time you do that same task because more is retained in your brain. With poor concentration the exact opposite is true—a task takes longer, may have mistakes, and the next time you do it you may still have difficulty remembering what you did right the first time. And this can lead to stress, which actually makes your concentration more difficult, and that all becomes a vicious cycle.

In addition to overwhelmingly busy lives, experts point to some other things that are definite "attention sappers." Lack of sleep, technology overload, and not getting enough exercise all make for difficulties in focus and attention.

Oxidative Stress and Free Radicals

But most important to cognitive difficulties, leading to both memory and concentration issues, is the damage done to cells by oxidative stress caused by free radicals. Oxidative stress is especially damaging to brain cells, or neurons, because human beings only have a limited amount of neurons.

They are the only cells in the body that cannot repair themselves, or are replaced by new ones. Once a brain cell dies, it is lost forever.

ESSENTIAL

Green tea has proven antioxidative power. Its catechins and polyphenols have many health benefits. There is also a better way to get green tea benefits than the average brewed teabag. It is called *matcha*. Matcha is powdered leaves of the green tea plant that are not brewed but dissolved in water for a drink with the power of the entire tea plant. It has been used as a healing elixir and in enlightening Buddhist ceremonies for centuries.

Recent scientific research suggests that a diet rich in antioxidants can help to preserve and protect brain cells from oxidative stress. In fact, one study conducted by the University of California proved that you could indeed teach an old dog new tricks—if you feed them the proper diet! In the study, seventy beagles were split into two groups and followed over several years of their lives. One group was fed a typical canine diet, the other a diet rich in plant source antioxidants. The dogs in the antioxidant group were able to perform and learn tasks much better than those fed the typical diet. Maybe even more noteworthy is that MRI scans of the brains of the dogs fed the antioxidant diet showed a lessening amount of the buildup of amyloid plaque. This is a goopy substance that forms around aging brain cells that is believed to be part of the development of the dreaded Alzheimer's disease.

FACT

Ginkgo biloba, from the root of the ginkgo tree, has been shown to improve memory and cognition. It not only has powerful antioxidants, which help to lower free radical damage to brain cells, but it is also believed that ginkgo opens up tiny blood vessels that feed oxygen to the brain.

Best Nutrients for Good Cognitive Function

You are not really using your brain to its full capacity—and most of the time it's because you are eating a diet and living a lifestyle that makes thinking clearly difficult. Cognition, memory, and "good ol' fashioned brain power" in general are all affected by the foods you eat.

Vitamin B, Again?

B complex vitamins are important to clear thinking, good memory, and cognitive function, especially vitamins B_{12} and B_6 and folic acid (B_9). Choline is a B complex vitamin found in eggs that has also been shown to improve alertness and mental sharpness. Alphabetically speaking you will also find anything from anthropology to zoology a little easier to understand by increasing vitamins A, E, and C, whose powerful antioxidant abilities protect brain cells.

ALERT

Finished carving that jack-o'-lantern on Halloween? If you want to scare off cognitive difficulties, don't throw away the seeds! Pumpkin is a super food, but the heart of its power is in those little seeds. Pumpkin seeds have many of the best known brain-building nutrients, including: vitamin A and E, zinc, and the vital omega-3 fatty acids. You can also get pumpkin seeds bagged in any season.

In addition to vitamins, there are a variety of minerals that help concentration and memory. The mental minerals and noggin nutrients include: calcium, potassium, magnesium, zinc, iron, and beta-carotene.

Here, Fishie

Fish has long been referred to as "brain food," and with good reason. Fish is high in omega-3 fatty acids. The cellular walls of neurons, or brain cells, that pass signals to one another and are responsible for thought and intelligence are mostly made up of fats. Studies have found that when the fatty membranes are made up mostly of omega-3 amino acids, they transmit signals better. The membranes are continually refreshed by fatty acids, so the more omega-3s the brain gets to make new membranes, the better the transmission and clearer the signals. Think of it this way: The difference in cell walls between a person who has enough omega-3s or other fatty acids and a person whose cell walls are *not* rich in those omega-3s is like the difference between a dial-up and a high-speed broadband Internet connection. Both will process information, but evidence points out which one will get it faster and more efficiently.

Sugar

The brain's main power supply is sugar. But don't go reaching for that candy bar just before an exam or that big presentation at work. The brain needs sugars and carbs, but not the processed kind. Those empty calories will leave you crashing and scratching your head, saying "huh?" The brain needs the complex carbohydrates and low-glycemic sugars found in whole grains, vegetables, legumes, fruits, and dairy products.

Fiber and Protein

On the subject of sugar metabolism and brain function, it is also important to consider fiber. Fiber metabolizes slowly, and it actually helps to lower the glycemic index of other foods and therefore it helps to keep a constant, steady supply of glucose in the blood to help brain function without spikes and crashes.

ESSENTIAL

Seeds such as flaxseed, sunflower seeds, and sesame seeds are great sources of cognitive compounds. These seeds are high in antioxidants as well as protein, vitamin E, and magnesium—all great neuro-nutrients.

Protein is important for good brain function and memory. Proteins are the sources of amino acids. Again, cognition, concentration, and memory all depend on communication between brain cells, which is done by neurotransmitters. Neurotransmitters are made up of essential amino acids, namely the amino acids tryptophan and tyrosine.

Superfoods

Many of the antioxidants found in the so-called "superfoods" have been linked to improvements in brain functions and memory.

ESSENTIAL

Deep-colored berries, blueberries, blackberries, and strawberries, have been linked to protecting brain cells and preventing cognitive difficulties. Recent studies have found that these berries may also improve the function of neurons that are already showing signs of not functioning properly and that have poor intercellular communication.

These include lycopene in tomatoes, ellagic acid in blueberries and blackberries, and the catechins and polyphenols in green tea. A compound called *phenylalanine* found in many nuts has been noted to add to brain functions. Almonds are high in both phenylalanine and vitamin E, making them a great brain-boosting snack.

What to Put in Your Shopping Cart

Here are some of the best nutrient rich foods that can help you with your cleanse. Choose as many as you can for your cleanse, and continue to choose them for use in your daily diet.

- **Vitamin A foods:** citrus fruit, tomatoes, carrots, mango, red bell pepper, spinach, collard greens, sweet potatoes, kale, turnip greens, Swiss chard, milk, and eggs
- **Vitamin B$_6$ foods:** tuna, cod, salmon, snapper, halibut, chicken, liver, turkey, beef, banana, spinach, bell pepper, turnip greens, garlic, cauliflower, mustard greens, cremini mushrooms, Brussels sprouts, cabbage, asparagus, celery, kale, Swiss chard, and collard greens
- **Vitamin B$_9$ (folic acid) foods:** liver, lentils, pinto beans, garbanzo beans, black beans, navy beans, asparagus, spinach, collard greens, broccoli, beets, romaine, parsley, papaya, and string beans
- **Vitamin B$_{12}$ foods:** fish, meat, poultry, eggs, and dairy products

- **Vitamin C foods:** bell peppers, parsley, broccoli, peppers, berries, citrus fruits, papaya, strawberries, cauliflower, mustard greens, spinach, snow peas, cantaloupe, watermelon, tomato, zucchini, and celery
- **Vitamin E foods:** mustard greens, chard, turnip greens, almonds, spinach, sunflower seeds, olives, papaya, and blueberries
- **Calcium foods:** spinach, turnip and mustard greens, collard greens, kale, molasses, Swiss chard, yogurt, milk, basil, thyme, dill, cinnamon, peppermint, and cheese
- **Beta-carotene foods:** sweet potatoes, carrots, kale, spinach, turnip greens, winter squash, collard greens, cilantro, thyme, cantaloupe, romaine, and broccoli
- **Magnesium foods:** beans, turmeric, spinach, squash, and mustard greens
- **Zinc foods:** liver, sea vegetables, pumpkin seeds, spinach, yeast, lamb, beef, summer squash, asparagus, Swiss chard, and wheat germ
- **Iron foods:** chard, spinach, thyme, turmeric, romaine, molasses, tofu, dill, parsley, basil, green beans, and wheat germ
- **Fiber foods/complex carbs/whole-grain foods:** fresh fruits, especially pears and apples, fresh vegetables, all whole grains, nuts, bran, flaxseeds, wheat germ, oats, brown rice, buckwheat, corn, millet, quinoa, and barley
- **Healthy fats, including omega-3s:** olive oil, flaxseed oil, flaxseeds, salmon, walnuts, sardines, halibut, snapper, soybeans, and tofu
- **Superfood antioxidants:** tomatoes, blueberries, blackberries, strawberries, raspberries, cherries, acai berries, black plums, orange, grapefruit, red grapes, and dark green leafy vegetables
- **Amino acid foods/tyrosine/tryptophan:** seafood, soy products, eggs, dairy, meat, tuna, snapper, halibut, beans, turkey, cremini mushrooms, bulgar wheat, oats, and brown rice
- **Herbs/teas:** green tea, sage, ginger, ginkgo, and unsweetened cacao with 86 percent dark chocolate

How a Cleanse Can Help

Your body may be up and working but your brain is functioning in slow motion. The real truth is a lack of certain nutrients and too much of the wrong stuff will slow a brain; conversely, all the right nutrients will feed the brain to a nice, healthy action. It's a drag to try to wish understanding to jump off a page when it just doesn't.

ESSENTIAL

The spice sage is an outstanding memory enhancer. Recent published studies prove what herbalists have known for years, that sage improves immediate recall and memory in general. The studies reported that sage has compounds like those in modern drugs that are being used for Alzheimer's. Add this aromatic herb to entrées, soups, and salads.

But there is a real path to take to clear out the debris and carve a path to clarity through that jungle, opening up your communication waves to your brain. By following the right nutrient path, beginning with a cleanse for better focus and concentration, you will be getting the right fuel to the right receptors and eliminating those that get in the way. Your brain will be helped to store what you want, and you will be helping your brain to pull out that information when you want it.

Begin your day with a large glass of water with a squirt of lemon or lime juice. Choose a breakfast, lunch, and dinner. Some recipes are suggested later in this chapter. Choose two snacks in between meals. One snack suggestion is a beverage blend of 1 cup water with ¼ cup tofu and add ½ banana or apple or pear, and 1 teaspoon of nut butter or sesame paste. For a cool drink, blend 1 or 2 ounces of watermelon, cantaloupe, or cucumber with water and ice. Be sure to drink eight to ten glasses of fluids a day, using teas and water. You may also choose to have hot chocolate with 1–2 tablespoons unsweetened cocoa and ¼ cup milk of choice. Sweeten with stevia. Aim to do your cleanse for one to three days.

After the Cleanse

Begin to increase your selection and amounts of solid foods. For a great interim meal, spread a slice of whole grain pita (or rice crackers) with 1 teaspoon of chickpea hummus, or use 1 teaspoon of a spread made from a mixture of ½ cup cooked navy beans, 1 teaspoon olive oil, ½ teaspoon sage, and 1 garlic clove. Top with a ½ can of mashed sardines or tuna, with a slice of tomato and sprinkle of flaxseed. Or, another meal choice is made with cooked buckwheat kernels, or roasted kasha. You can make a fabulous pilaf with it by adding in any combinations of vegetables, fruits, nuts, or chicken. Or, cut up and roast an eggplant, onion, and garlic, season with thyme, and combine with garbanzos, sesame tahini, feta cheese, and walnuts.

ALERT

The brain is a glutton for carbs. In fact the brain uses 20 percent of the body's whole carbohydrate supply. The brain uses carbohydrates for fuel, and with a steady and constant supply of sugar, it moves along nice and clear. But when levels of sugar in the blood go up and down sharply like they do with a diet that is high in processed and other high-glycemic foods, the brain doesn't get its steady fuel supply; instead, it sputters and starts and stops like a car with clogged fuel injectors.

Remember that there are many wonderful and nutritious foods you can choose from that will help to keep your body and head healthy today, and every day. Using a wide variety of foods in your everyday diet is the way to take the best and the most of what the earth has to offer.

- Keep your drinking/flushing habits alive with herbal teas and water.
- Do some exercise—both cardio and strength training. Aim for four times a week, and walk every day. Exercise releases endorphins, which enhance neurotransmitters and clear your head.
- Stretching is important. It increases oxygen and blood flow, and decreases stress.

By making the right nutrition choices you will think clearer, remember more, and will have given yourself some real food for thought.

Oatmeal Old-Fashioned Beverage

This recipe involves about twelve hours' pre-preparation, so keep that in mind. Put ¼ cup of oats in a bowl of water before you go to bed, and they will be ready to rock and roll the next morning.

INGREDIENTS | **YIELDS 1 SERVING**

¼ cup rolled oats just barely covered with water, soaked overnight

1 cup berries of your choice

1–2 pitted dried prunes

2 teaspoons honey

2 tablespoons toasted wheat germ

1 teaspoon ground flaxseed

½ cup fat free soy, rice, or almond milk

1 (2-ounce) scoop protein powder

1 cup water

1. Add the soaked oats to a blender with any remaining water, and blend.

2. Add all the remaining ingredients and blend until smooth.

Asparagus Simply Soup

This recipe requires some pre-preparation. Soak your macadamia and pine nuts in water overnight, and they will be ready to go the next day. You can also enjoy this soup raw and cold by not steaming the vegetables and cooling or omitting the rice.

INGREDIENTS | YIELDS 4 SERVINGS

½ cup chopped onion or green onion

1 tablespoon extra-virgin olive oil

1 stalk finely chopped celery

1 pound asparagus, trimmed of hard ends and chopped small (about 1½ cups)

⅓ cup jasmine or basmati rice, uncooked

1 sprig thyme or 1 teaspoon dry

1 sprig fresh parsley

4 cups broth or water

¼ cup macadamia nuts soaked overnight and drained

¼ cup pine nuts soaked overnight and drained

1. In a skillet over medium heat, sauté the onion in olive oil until soft, about 3–4 minutes.

2. Add all the other ingredients and simmer 30 minutes, or until the rice is tender.

3. Let cool, and carefully add to a blender in batches; purée until smooth.

Brain Broccoli Soup

This recipe contains walnuts, which have long been called a brain food for their nutrients.

INGREDIENTS | YIELDS 1–2 SERVINGS

2 cups broccoli florets

1 tablespoon extra-virgin olive oil

⅓ cup walnuts soaked to soften overnight

½ cup basil or parsley

1 cup spinach, roughly chopped

½ clove garlic

1 tablespoon lemon or lime juice (optional)

1 anchovy fillet

1½ cups vegetable stock or water

¼ cup plain, nonfat yogurt (optional)

1. Steam the broccoli in water about 3–4 minutes, or microwave for 1 minute.

2. Add the steamed broccoli to a blender along with all the other ingredients and blend until smooth.

3. Serve warm or cold with yogurt swirled in if desired.

Sultry Salmon Soup

Salmon is one of the best sources you can find of omega-3s. Omega-3s are necessary for serotonin, a key neurotransmitter. Not enough serotonin is a cause of depression, anxiety, and forgetfulness.

INGREDIENT | YIELDS 4 SERVINGS

½ cup chopped onion
½ cup chopped green bell pepper
½ cup chopped celery
½ cup chopped carrots
½ cup large-diced sweet or white potato
1 garlic clove
1 tablespoon extra-virgin olive oil
2 cups vegetable broth
½ teaspoon dill
Sea salt and pepper, to taste
1 (5-ounce) can salmon
¼ cup plain, nonfat yogurt

1. In a large skillet over medium heat, sauté the onion, bell pepper, celery, carrots, potato, and garlic in the olive oil about 4 minutes.

2. Add the broth and seasonings and simmer about 30 minutes.

3. Stir in salmon, and just heat about 2–3 minutes.

4. Let cool, and add to a blender. Blend carefully in batches until smooth. Swirl in yogurt to serve.

Peasing Avocado Cold or Warm Soup

Green peas are an excellent source of Vitamin B_1, which is essential for memory function.

INGREDIENTS | YIELDS 2–3 SERVINGS

¾ cup frozen peas

1 avocado

2 cups vegetable stock or water

2 green onions, chopped

2 teaspoons lemon or lime juice

½ cup chopped cherry tomatoes

½ cup chopped spinach

1 teaspoon extra-virgin olive oil

2 teaspoons ground flaxseed

2 tablespoons chopped cilantro, or to taste

½ cup soaked walnuts (or almonds, or sunflower seeds), ground

2 tablespoons plain, nonfat Greek-style or soy yogurt, or 2 tablespoons grated Parmesan cheese

1. Blend all the ingredients, except yogurt or Parmesan cheese, in a blender until smooth.

2. Swirl in the yogurt or Parmesan to taste to serve. You may also warm this soup if you wish.

CHAPTER 14

Cleansing for Calm, Balance, Homeostasis

The phrase "don't worry, be happy" is often used, and was even part of a popular song. The message behind that phrase is to be upbeat, easy going, and forget about rushing along. But that is a state of being that many people find difficult to achieve because they often find themselves under pressure and constrained for time. And that all makes for stress and tension. The tensing up that you can see in your mirror is not only a reflection of your outer appearance but your inner body processes as well. When you're tight and stressed it can be difficult to "not worry and be happy" and you can wind up on a downward spiral of the blues. But cheer up, because studies have indicated there are many nutrients you can easily find in foods that can break that vicious cycle, and work on the body's processes to help you feel better, improve mood, and return a state of balance and calm.

Typical Stress Issues

The ability to be able to gather yourself together with a deep breath (or even with a four-letter word) and let it go—to do whatever it takes to come back to a place where you can feel balanced—is critical to your health and happiness.

Mind Over Matter

You can get on the path to having that calm, balance, or homeostasis, beginning with a cleanse with nutrients aimed at working toward what your body needs to avoid feeling out-of-whack and stressed. Ancient philosophers and even modern Western medicine now agree that there really is a mind/body connection when it comes to health and wellness.

ESSENTIAL

Feeling a little down in the dumps? The omega-3s in walnuts are one of the world's greatest natural antidepressants. Or, do you have a quick temper? Maybe you are not getting enough B vitamins. Vitamin B$_6$ has been shown to curb feelings of anger and aggression.

The concept of the mind/body connection is the basis for the spiritual beliefs and healing philosophies of Taoism, Reiki, yoga, traditional Chinese medicine, and many others. And, there is undeniable scientific evidence that mental and emotional states do affect your physical health. It is well documented that blood pressure rises with stress and anxiety. A recent report from the American Academy of Family Physicians, *How Your Emotions Affect Your Health*, states: "our bodies react to the way we feel, think, and act, and respond accordingly." Basically that means when you feel anxious, stressed-out, or upset, the body will often respond with a physical issue. And so, the report lists the following issues or conditions as ones that can all be caused by emotional stress:

- Back pain
- Chest pain
- Fibromyalgia

- Gastric distress
- General body aches
- Chronic pain
- Head pain
- High blood pressure

Not all stress is bad; in fact, stress is one of your body's defenses. When you are put in a stressful situation, the body goes into a state of extra alertness—hormones and chemicals make muscles tense up and get ready for action. This what is called the "fight-or-flight reaction." Today many people are in a state of constant stress just because of the nature of modern life, and not because they are being chased by a tiger! The problem is, when you have such constant pressure, the body never relaxes from that state of "fight or flight" and many physical and emotional problems are the result.

ESSENTIAL

People have long considered chocolate a "comfort food," and recent clinical research seems to indicate that it can improve mood. But not the sugary milk chocolate found in typical candy bars. A study published by the American Chemical Society found that eating about 1½ ounces of dark chocolate a day for two weeks reduced the levels of stress-related hormones in the bodies of individuals in the study who considered themselves "highly stressed." Dark chocolate, with at least 70 percent cocoa content, is also known to be high in antioxidants.

Don't Stress Out!

Not putting the best combinations of nutrients into your body adds to the body's level of stress with any or all of the above issues, and it can lead to depression as well. But you can help beat the blues by what you do or do not put in your belly. That anxious feeling often described as "frayed nerves" actually could be your body reacting to not getting what it wants in certain vitamins, minerals, or other nutrients that really do keep nerves transmitting their signals back and forth to each other properly.

Often when in a state of being "stressed out," it's easy to make food choices that may not be the best. In running late for that 9 A.M. meeting, you grab a breakfast "no-no" at the drive-through, or, if alone and sleepless, worrying about this, that, or the other, you reach for the comfort of that chocolate cake and gallon of ice cream. When times get tough, food can be your best friend or worst enemy; it's all about the choices you make.

Best Nutrients for Fighting Stress

Taking care of everything you need to juggle in a day can often seem monumental. And that all leads to one thing: stress. But fortunately there are some good and positive ways to combat that stress—with a trip to the grocery store. There are many foods that can be added to your diet to reduce stress, anxiety, and depression, and return your body to both physical, as well as emotional, balance.

ALERT

Feeling down during the winter months? According to medical experts it may not just be a case of the "holiday blues." There is an actual condition known as seasonal affective disorder (SAD), and it can be prevented with diet. Two important neurotransmitters that affect mood are serotonin and melatonin, and levels of sunlight either help or limit these chemicals. During a long dark winter, these chemicals can be reduced so much that depression can result. But the good news is a diet rich in magnesium and good carbs from veggies and omega-3s can boost the serotonin and melatonin.

Vitamin B for the Blues

Vitamins might be one thing you think of if your body *needs* something. The family of B complex vitamins has been found to be great blues busters. Vitamin B_1 can improve mood states and is essential for stable nerve transmissions. Vitamin B_3 is critical to help regulate sleep patterns; lack of sleep is a major factor in stress and anxiety. Serotonin is a neurotransmitter, or brain chemical. It is the neurotransmitter most responsible for mood. Antidepressant medications work to regulate the level of serotonin. Vitamin B_6 can do the same thing without the harmful side effects of such mood-altering drugs. Vitamin B_5, also known as pantothenic acid, helps the hormones put out by the adrenal glands, which controls the body's fight-or-flight reaction to stress. Vitamin B_{12} is also important in making serotonin and dopamine, another one of the brain's "feel good" chemicals. B_{12} is also essential for melatonin, the chemical that helps our sleep/wakefulness cycle. Choline is a B vitamin found in eggs that has been found to reduce anxiety.

Vitamin A helps to get rid of toxins that cause weakness and fatigue and that can often lead to depression. Vitamin E is a powerful antioxidant that can fight the buildup of oxidative stress in the brain. This oxidative stress can lower serotonin and dopamine, which causes depression, anxiety, and other troublesome moods. During times of stress the body uses up vitamin C, so lower levels of vitamin C can lead to feelings of nervousness and irritability.

Calcium, Chromium, and Magnesium

Equally as important as vitamins to staying calm and keeping moods more balanced are certain minerals. Calcium, chromium, and magnesium all can reduce stress, help you to relax, and stabilize blood sugar levels. Selenium helps vitamin E in its antioxidant work. Zinc helps in resistance to infection, and when you aren't coming down with some infection you are less apt to feel stress. Omega-3 amino acids are believed to help neurotransmitters to get through cell membranes, which means they can help lessen irritability and help to fight anxiety and depression.

Important neurotransmitters need the amino acid tryptophan. Increasing your intake of tryptophan can boost the levels of the feel-good chemicals and the chemicals that regulate sleep. Protein is necessary for the amino acids needed for all the brain chemicals that influence mood.

Your brain needs carbohydrates to provide sugar for fuel. But too many processed carbs leads to spikes and valleys in glucose levels in the blood, which makes for mood swings. Complex carbs from whole grains and veggies are useful so that sugar levels, and thus moods, will keep more constant.

Nutritional chemicals called *adaptogens* have been found to lower cortisol levels. Cortisol is what triggers the adrenal glands to put out adrenaline and other fight-or-flight chemicals in stressful situations. Interestingly enough, adaptogens that have this tranquilizing effect are found in ginseng, kava, and licorice—all roots that were used for centuries to create teas or "calming tonics" long before the discovery of the adaptogenic compounds.

FACT

Theanine is an amino acid that binds with certain brain chemicals and in doing so has a calming and stress-reducing effect. Theanine is highly present in the leaves of green tea, and may account for the soothing effect reported by green tea drinkers. So curl up and relax with a glass of green tea; besides the theanine, knowing you are doing your body good with the antioxidants alone should be enough to ease your mind.

The foods that contain these vital vitamins, minerals, amino acids, and other nutrients are the true "comfort foods." When feeling down, look for them, and avoid reaching for energy drinks, the empty calories of candy bars, and other trans-fat laden junk foods, caffeinated beverages, or alcohol.

What to Put in Your Shopping Cart

Here are some of the best nutrient-rich foods that can help you with your cleanse. Choose as many of them as you can for your cleanse and keep choosing from these foods for use in your daily diet.

- **Vitamin A foods:** citrus fruit, tomatoes, carrots, mango, red bell pepper, spinach, collard greens, sweet potatoes, kale, turnip greens, Swiss chard, milk, and eggs
- **Vitamin B$_1$ (thiamin) foods:** asparagus, romaine, mushrooms, spinach, sunflower seeds, celery, tuna, green peas, tomatoes, eggplant, Brussels sprouts, celery, and watermelon

- **Vitamin B$_3$ (niacin) foods:** chicken, tuna, salmon, mushrooms, liver, halibut, lamb, turkey, cremini mushrooms, sardines, and asparagus
- **Vitamin B$_5$ foods:** liver, cauliflower, mushrooms, sunflower seeds, cremini mushrooms, corn, yogurt, broccoli, squash, and eggs
- **Vitamin B$_6$ foods:** tuna, cod, salmon, snapper, halibut, chicken, liver, turkey, beef, banana, spinach, bell peppers, turnip greens, garlic, cauliflower, mustard greens, cremini mushrooms, Brussels sprouts, cabbage, asparagus, celery, kale, Swiss chard, and collard greens
- **Vitamin B$_9$ (folic acid) foods:** liver, lentils, pinto beans, garbanzo beans, black beans, navy beans, asparagus, spinach, collard greens, broccoli, beets, romaine, parsley, papaya, and string beans
- **Vitamin B$_{12}$ foods:** fish, meat, poultry, eggs, and dairy products
- **Vitamin C foods:** bell peppers, parsley, broccoli, peppers, berries, citrus fruits, papaya, strawberries, cauliflower, mustard greens, spinach, snow peas, cantaloupe, watermelon, tomatoes, zucchini, and celery
- **Vitamin E foods:** mustard greens, Swiss chard, turnip greens, almonds, spinach, sunflower seeds, olives, papaya, and blueberries
- **Calcium foods:** spinach, turnip and mustard greens, collard greens, kale, molasses, Swiss chard, yogurt, milk, basil, thyme, dill, cinnamon, peppermint, and cheese
- **Chromium foods:** romaine, onion, tomatoes, Brewer's yeast, oysters, liver, whole grains, grain, and potatoes
- **Magnesium and folate foods:** beans, turmeric, corn, spinach, squash, mustard greens, pumpkin, soybeans, sunflower seeds, flaxseeds, sesame seeds, green beans, cucumbers, celery, kale, black and navy beans, peppermint, and molasses
- **Zinc foods:** liver, sea vegetables, pumpkin seeds, spinach, yeast, lamb, beef, summer squash, asparagus, Swiss chard, wheat germ, brewer's yeast
- **Selenium foods:** liver, Brazil nuts, snapper, cod, halibut, tuna, salmon, sardines, shrimp, barley, oats, mushrooms, sunflower seeds, eggs, turkey, lamb, tofu, and wheat germ
- **Healthy fats, including omega-3s:** olive oil, flaxseed oil, flaxseeds, salmon, walnuts, sardines, halibut, snapper, soybeans, and tofu

- **Foods with amino acid tryptophan:** wheat germ, cottage cheese, eggs, duck, turkey, granola, chicken, black-eyed peas, walnuts, almonds, sesame seeds, Swiss and Gruyère cheese, shrimp, tamari, cremini mushrooms, cod, tuna, snapper, halibut, mustard greens, spinach, tofu, banana, beef liver, sardines, salmon, soybeans, mustard seeds, cauliflower, black beans, kidney beans, and milk
- **Complex carbs:** bananas, beans, oats, lentils, barley, brown rice, buckwheat, wheat germ, bran, whole wheat, chickpeas, nuts, seeds, potatoes, corn, peas, root vegetables, yams, parsnips, whole-grain breads, cereals, pasta, fruits such as apricots, oranges, grapefruits, prunes, pears, and most vegetables
- **Proteins:** lean meat, poultry, fish, eggs, dairy, soy products, nuts, seeds, and beans
- **Herbs/teas:** green tea, cloves, cinnamon, nutmeg, ginger, ginseng, and unsweetened cocoa

ALERT

The things many people turn to when stressed out often add to the problem—the easily metabolized carbs in surgary and salty snacks, white breads, and processed cereals can cause the release of the stress hormone cortisol. Stimulants such as coffee, nicotine, and alcohol give a temporary and false emotional boost, lead to later crashes, and can put the body under additional stress.

How a Cleanse Can Help

The street of stress is often hard to get off of. Even if you know all about how yoga, meditation, deep breathing, or simply taking time for yourself can reduce stress, you may not always find the time to do what you know is good for you. Finding that right stress-reducing hobby, technique, or activity may be different for each person, but for any type of personality, eating the right foods may be the one universal truth. Leaving behind the foods and beverages that may actually be a contributing factor to your stress and taking a cleanse that will put you on the path to getting the nutrients you need for happier feelings, avoiding feeling stress, and for feeling a balance about things, can work for anybody. Aim to do your cleanse for one to three days.

Begin your day with a large glass of water with a squirt of lemon or lime juice and a teaspoon of ground flaxseed. Choose a breakfast, lunch, and dinner. Some recipes are suggested later in this chapter. Choose two snacks in between meals. One snack suggestion is a beverage blend of 1 cup water, ¼ cup tofu, ½ banana or apple or pear, and 1 teaspoon of nut butter or sesame paste. Or, for a cool drink, blend a handful of watermelon or cucumber chunks with water and ice. Celery juice is a traditional remedy for nervous tension. Blend up a good stalk or two of celery with water and ice, and drink whenever you wish.

Be sure to drink eight to ten glasses of fluids a day, using teas and water. You may also choose to have a hot chocolate with 1–2 tablespoons unsweetened cocoa, and ¼–½ cup milk of your choice. Sweeten with stevia, honey, or pure maple syrup.

ESSENTIAL

Skipping breakfast is never a good idea; it can put you into an unpleasant mood until lunch. For a real good morning, start the day off with a balanced breakfast including complex carbs and protein. You'll not only give your brain a needed positive energy boost, but you will be less irritable and subject to food cravings.

You can add a sprig of mint leaves or slice of ginger or lemon to your green tea, or a splash of juice—pineapple or cranberry. Or, add a little hot soy or almond milk and spice it up with cinnamon, allspice, ginger, and pepper. A fresh rosemary tea can be made with a rosemary sprig soaked in a cup of hot water for about 10–15 minutes. Strain and add stevia or honey to sweeten. The scent of rosemary has long been used in aromatherapy for its calming and soothing effect. Using the spice in foods can lower the levels of cortisol, a stress hormone that pumps out fight-or-flight chemicals from the adrenal glands. Rosemary also seems to boost brain chemicals responsible for clear thinking and memory.

A traditional home remedy for a relaxing sleep is to heat ½ cup milk, ½ cup water, and a spoon of molasses. Molasses is rich in B complex for fighting stress as well as other minerals including iron and magnesium.

After the Cleanse

Basically, the recommendations for continuing to fight stress are five servings of fruit and vegetables per day, three servings of dairy products a day, three servings of grains a day for fiber, and one to two servings of protein.

You might start off with a snack of crunchy veggies or whole-grain baked chips with a whipped asparagus pesto dip. Just purée some asparagus, garlic, and Parmesan cheese, and add a little olive oil and seasonings to taste. Spread a slice of whole-grain pita with 1 teaspoon of chickpea hummus, or use 1 teaspoon of a spread made from a mixture of ½ cup cooked navy beans, 1 teaspoon olive oil, ½ teaspoon sage, and 1 garlic clove. Top with a ½ can of mashed sardines or tuna, a slice of tomato, and a sprinkle of flaxseed. Or, make a fabulous pilaf with cooked buckwheat kernels, or roasted kasha combined with any vegetables, fruits, nuts, or chicken. Or, cut up and roast an eggplant, onion, and garlic, season with thyme, and combine with garbanzos, sesame tahini, feta cheese, and walnuts.

The choices of nutritious foods are almost limitless—especially when you think of the combinations possible. Health professionals all agree that optimal health comes from eating a wide variety of foods to get the benefits of the many types of nutrients. Always remember the necessity of fluids—so keep your drinking/flushing habits alive with herbal teas and water. In addition to treating yourself to great nutrients, add some stress-relieving activities to your schedule. Plan to try for two or three of these a week. At least give each one of them a shot to see how you like the effects.

Anytime you are in a real rush and want a quick, healthy, easy, antistress food, think of these possible choices: a banana, baked tortilla chips and salsa, a bowl of oatmeal and spiced apples, black bean soup, whole-grain raisin bread with farmer or cottage cheese, a decaf nonfat latte, or baby carrots with yogurt dip with herbs or spices of your choice.

By making the right nutrition choices you will give your body what it needs to remain calm and stress free, and you will find that more than your diet will be balanced.

Move Your Body

Physical exercise is truly effective for relieving stress. Aerobic exercise works so well because it changes your body chemistry—it helps release those endorphins that can put you in an overall better state and mood. Yoga and tai chi are traditional exercises that use certain poses, moves, and breathing that goes along with the moves. Strength training also benefits, and often both cardio and strength training combined work together to release endorphins that help those neurotransmitters in your head work toward relieving stress. Aim for three or four times a week, and walk at least a little every day.

Stretching is also important. It increases oxygen and blood flow, and decreases stress.

Breathing is always one of the first recommendations to avoid or deal with stress and anxiety. One of the breathing patterns that is used in some yoga is done to help you feel a balance with the world. In this technique you sit straight and breathe in deeply for a count of eight seconds. Don't breathe out yet, but push your stomach out for a count of four seconds, then for another two seconds feel your rib cage midsection lifting up; then for a count of two seconds, lift up your chest and neck. Still try to hold your breath for two more seconds, then let it out slowly for eight seconds.

Meditation is often used for relaxation and stopping tension. A certain word or sound is often used to keep meditation going. Visualizing some particular loved or precious object or thing to focus on is another method. Or, you can imagine that you are a big, strong tree, with roots deep and firm in the earth, solid with branches that simply sway with any wind of tension. Meditation, like anything else, becomes easier and more a part of routine the more it is practiced.

Getting in touch with where your muscles tense can help. In this exercise, while lying down, you slowly elevate and lower parts of the body, breathing slowly in and out. You can tense up and release certain muscles—you get them working and then you give them their due release. This will get energy flowing throughout the tensed muscles, getting rid of wastes and stimulating good energy.

This may sound hilarious, but you can really shrink and erase your tensions. In this technique, you sit or lie down comfortably and do a little slow breathing. You take that stressful or tense situation or person and put it right there in your mind, and then you just tell your mind to shrink it. You might even hold out your hand and see that stressing picture shrinking down to fit in your palm until it is so tiny, it disappears. These techniques give you power, and so give you a sense of calm and mastery.

Color Me Relaxed

Stress can be relieved through color—just as you choose red, orange, and green fruits and veggies, certain colors have been noted by health professionals to be great for visualization. Research has supported the use of color and light for health, balance, emotions, and well-being. Colors and light can stimulate the immune system, nervous system, and endocrine glands. Some techniques use a particular color stone to focus and meditate on.

Blue is a particular tension releaser—a cool color of the sky that is expansive and in a way, airy and weightless. One technique is to sit comfortably, taking deep breaths, while filling your mind with the color blue, filling your whole body with the color blue. Similarly, the color red is often used to energize to combat stress-provoked tiredness.

Adding a daily note of affirmation on your morning mirror or fridge helps many to begin the day with a good mood and attitude. Such notes can be spiritual or religious passages, if you like, or poems or jokes. Affirmations are often a little statement about something you love about yourself to keep up your self-esteem no matter what comes along. It can be helpful to repeat an affirmation either to yourself or out loud for a few minutes.

Other Stress Busters

Sound is often helpful for nervous tension. Just as oftentimes the outside noise of traffic and industry makes for stress, taking some time to listen to music—especially quiet classics or nature sounds, can slow the heart rate, lower blood pressure and stress hormones, and help with sleep.

Hot baths or steaming showers are often helpful, meditative, and calming. Heat helps to release muscle tension, which also helps mood.

Plan to do whatever combination of stress-relieving exercises that work for you every day, if possible. Just twenty to thirty minutes a day will do you wonders.

Morning Slurp for Stress

This recipe will have you up and for your day before your alarm clock even has the chance to beep!

INGREDIENTS | YIELDS 1–2 SERVINGS

1 cup fresh or frozen berries

½ banana

1 tablespoon almond butter

½ cup orange juice

1 teaspoon ground flaxseeds

2 tablespoons toasted wheat germ

1 cup romaine or spinach

1½ cups water

Ice cubes, if desired

1 (2-ounce) scoop protein powder

1 dried, pitted date or prune

1 teaspoon honey or stevia to sweeten (optional)

1. Add all the ingredients to a blender and blend until smooth. Pour into a glass and serve.

2. Alternatively, substitute ½ cup tofu for the protein powder, and cantaloupe, mango, pear, or peaches, for the berries.

Creamy Easy Corn Soup

Corn is a food often overlooked for its nutritional value, but it is actually very high in pantothenic acid, a B vitamin most important in good adrenal gland function and stress reduction.

INGREDIENTS | YIELDS 1–2 SERVINGS

2 cups corn kernels (frozen or fresh)

3 green onions, chopped

1 stalk celery, chopped

1 teaspoon basil

1 tablespoon extra-virgin olive oil

1 cup broth of your choice

1 cup milk

Salt and pepper, to taste (optional)

⅓ can drained tuna, shrimp, or salmon (optional alternative)

1. In a medium skillet over medium heat, sauté the corn, green onions, celery, and basil in the olive oil for 5 minutes.

2. Add the broth and simmer for 5 minutes; add the milk and seasonings.

3. Let cool, and carefully blend in a blender in batches until smooth. Can be enjoyed cold as well as warm.

4. To make seafood bisque, add ⅓ cup drained canned shrimp, tuna, or salmon to the mixture before simmering.

Apple Peanut Butter Soup

The apple contains nutrients that can prevent and fight off germs that cause colds and other sicknesses.

INGREDIENTS | YIELDS 2–3 SERVINGS

1 chopped apple

¼ cup finely chopped celery

¼ cup chopped carrot

¼ cup chopped onion

1 tablespoon extra-virgin olive oil

2 cups milk, heated but not boiled (fat free or low fat, soy, rice, almond)

6 tablespoons peanut butter

Salt and pepper, to taste

Worcestershire sauce, to taste (optional)

Honey, to taste (optional)

1. In a large skillet over medium heat, sauté the apple, celery, carrot, and onion in the olive oil until tender, about 4 minutes.

2. Add to the blender. Add the milk, peanut butter, and seasonings and honey and Worcestershire if desired. Blend together in small batches until well mixed. May be served warm, or chill and enjoy cold.

Hidden Chocolate Soup

*The chocolate used in this recipe is unsweetened cocoa,
which you can buy at any supermarket or grocery store.*

INGREDIENTS | YIELDS 5 SERVINGS

2 tablespoons extra-virgin olive oil

2 tablespoons chopped sweet onion

1½ cups pureed roasted sweet red peppers

½ cup peanut butter

1 (15-ounce) can black beans, rinsed and drained

½ cup mushrooms

1 cup corn kernels

⅓ cup raisins

5 cups vegetable stock

2 tablespoons unsweetened cocoa

1 teaspoon ground cumin

1 teaspoon chili powder

1 teaspoon ground allspice

2 ounces (68 percent or higher) dark chocolate

⅓ cup soaked and ground almonds

½ cup low-fat, plain Greek-style or soy yogurt

1. In a medium skillet over medium heat, sauté the onions in oil for about 2 minutes. Reduce heat to low and add the red pepper purée, peanut butter, beans, mushrooms, corn, raisins, stock, cocoa, and spices; cook for about 5 minutes.

2. Let sit until cool enough to handle, and swirl in the dark chocolate. Blend carefully in small batches in a blender. For each serving, swirl in 1–2 teaspoons ground almonds and about 1 tablespoon yogurt.

Balancing Gazpacho Soup

You can mix and match with other important vegetables for stress: ½ cup shredded beets, ½ cup grated zucchini, 1 tablespoon cider vinegar or lemon juice, ¼ cup ground and blended pine nuts or pecans, and/ or increase or decrease amounts of vegetables according to taste.

INGREDIENTS | YIELDS 1 SERVING

1 cucumber, chopped

1 cup frozen cut green beans, thawed and chopped

2 stalks celery, without strings, chopped

1 tomato, chopped

¼ sweet onion, diced

½ green or red bell pepper, chopped

½ avocado

½–1 clove garlic, minced

½ cup parsley or basil

½ apple

1 teaspoon sea salt

Black pepper, to taste

1 teaspoon extra-virgin olive oil

1 teaspoon ground flaxseed

1 cup water

Optional herbs to taste: sage, rosemary, thyme, oregano

Blend all ingredients in a food processor or blender until smooth and serve.

CHAPTER 15

Post-Cleanse: Keeping Good Habits and Ending Your Cleanse—Safely

You did it! In doing your cleanse, the rules are for you to make to keep yourself safe at all times. You always succeed by putting forth the effort and trying to bring yourself to a healthier place, no matter how small the increments. Just by counting yourself in, you will accomplish your goals at your own safe speed. If you need to stop and rest and resume another time, that's okay. Always make sure you are eating and drinking enough. Many times with new foods you need to try them out. If a food doesn't work for you, try another or take something easy, familiar, and healthy like a banana, apple, brown rice, whole-grain pasta, or 100 percent fruit or vegetable juice.

Transitioning Back into a Normal Diet

When your cleanse comes to an end you might take an attitude of looking at the positive stuff that you gained. Sure, there may always be goals or expectations you had that weren't achieved. But more likely what is learned and achieved will outweigh areas that weren't—and when it comes to health, you have your whole life to make it work well for you. *By no means should you continue your cleanse longer than the recommended time for any reason.*

QUESTION

Why is breakfast so important?
If you've ever stopped to look at the word, you'll see the answer right there for you: "break fast." Breaking the fast after sleeping is the most important health and nutritional boost you can give your body. Skipping breakfast will slow your metabolism and put your body into a dull, slow hibernation mode. You need to fuel up for the day with healthy whole foods to be physically strong and mentally awake to deal with your morning and late afternoon grind.

When you do start to get back into a regular eating routine, that is the time to make a few changes in what might be "regular" and "routine" for you. Both Western and Eastern health practices would agree that there are some eating habits that really work well for digestion and health. They can be easily seen as five tips:

1. Eat three to six smaller meals a day. Make sure breakfast is the first one!
2. Recommendations are often for a lighter meal in the evening, with the more substantial, larger meals at breakfast and lunch.
3. Ayurvedic guidelines offer these wonderful suggestions for meals at home: eat in a lovely atmosphere, pay attention to the food you eat, chew slowly to allow mouth digestive juices to work, and enjoy pleasant conversation during the meal.
4. Eastern traditions also recommend a minute of quiet sitting before you begin eating. This is similar to the old tradition of saying grace before

a meal. Relaxing for a minute or two after finishing a meal gives your digestion a chance to begin.

5. An old guideline for determining the amount to eat is to think of ¾ of your stomach capacity. Your stomach capacity is usually compared to the size of your fist! That's not too big!

Don't Backslide!

When you finish a cleanse, it can be an interesting moment to consider what your food faults are. How or when or what do you eat that you now see is contributing to any health issues? Just take note of them, and say to yourself, "okay, this is what I'm going to do about that"; then make some kind of plan to deal with that fault however many days of the week you decide to focus on it. Every little step forward counts—but, of course you know all that!

QUESTION

Why is protein so important?
Protein is made up of amino acids. Amino acids are the building blocks of everything vital to your body's healthy functioning. Neurotransmitters and anti-inflammatory, disease-fighting enzymes are made from amino acids. Protein provides the raw materials for health! There are a total of twenty important amino acids that make up the long-chain protein molecules. There are twelve that the body cannot make on its own; they must be obtained from the foods you eat. Good protein sources of these essential amino acids are nuts, seeds, and greens.

Many people do not pay attention to fiber in their diet. Some easy ways to add fiber is to add some fresh fruit, bran cereals, wheat germ or other healthy granolas to yogurt or cottage cheese. If you're making a casserole or soup, add beans, or oatmeal, or okra. When you are eating out, now that you know more about ingredients, you can make good or better choices. When you go shopping, read food labels. Often things are in tiny print; so, if you need reading glasses, bring them with you when you shop!

If portion size is a downfall, go gradually. You don't want to ever feel deprived; you know what that leads to! For a visual idea of portion size, about 3 ounces of cooked meat is the size of a deck of cards. One cup of something is about the size of a baseball. If you want larger portions in a meal, try adding more vegetables, beans, and fruits! But do forgive yourself if you make mistakes, because we all do.

Maintaining Balance

Some people have found success by allowing themselves one meal or one or two days a week to indulge in less healthy foods—keeping up the efforts during the other days. Denying yourself foods you enjoy entirely is a recipe for disaster; this is the number one surefire way to make sure you break your healthy habits. Moderation is key; you'll be surprised to see that one or two cookies, not the whole box, can satisfy your craving for sweets. Don't beat yourself up for wanting to partake in these foods, but make sure you moderate.

ESSENTIAL

We all know what junk foods are, and why they have that name—and yet they seem the hardest to avoid for many of us. But those cravings are not necessarily your fault. Years of a diet crammed with processed foods have rewired the brains of most Americans to crave these foods. You can reprogram your appetite by adding a few new fruits and vegetables to each meal and going for celery sticks or carrots instead of the bag of chips when craving the crunch.

Make up and plan for your own quick snack packets for take-alongs or easy fridge grabbing. Have fruits, yogurts, and trail mixes on hand. There are many easy recipes for raw, healthy granola bars you can make with your own favorite combinations. Supermarkets sell small baggies that are ideal for these quick snacks.

Be Good to Yourself

Give yourself some kind of weekly reward, whatever it is that pleases you—new clothing, a massage, one hour of family time, or whatever you like. But whatever it is, your efforts deserve some recognition! It is not easy to overhaul your diet after a cleanse, and you deserve something special for your hard work.

ALERT

Try to find a local farmer's market in your area. These markets feature produce and products from local farmers like fruits, veggies, and baked goods, and are often grown without pesticides. Several also continue indoors in the winter! You'll be benefiting local commerce and getting fresh and delicious produce for you and your family!

Foods to Avoid, Foods to Embrace

The healthy food pyramid, which traditionally listed amounts of servings of various food groups one should eat daily, has now branched out into several various types of recommended food pyramids. They have been devised to connect with various cultures and lifestyles, weight, and health concerns such as diabetics. They all report similar amounts to the following:

- **Carbs:** 4–8 daily servings, which includes 3 ounces of whole grains a day (1 ounce is equal to approximately 1 slice of bread, ½ cup cooked pasta, rice, or cereal, or 1 cup dry cereal)
- **Protein/dairy:** (this includes fish, poultry, beef, eggs, dairy, nuts, seeds, beans, and peas) 4–8 daily servings, or 5–5 ½ ounces a day
- **Fruits and vegetables:** a minimum of 3 fruits and 4 vegetables daily, or 2–4 servings of fruits daily and 2½–3 cups of vegetables a day.
- **Fats:** 3–5 daily servings, or 5–7 teaspoons per day

Whole Foods and Going Organic

Try to eat whole foods, as natural as when they come out of the earth, and avoid processed foods, preservatives, and other food additives such as artificial colors, flavors, and sweeteners.

Supermarkets now have natural and organic sections. Try to select some of your produce from these sections. Or, if you can buy local produce, that is often fresher, and not subject to agricultural processing such as chemicals and pesticides, radiating, long storage, and gas ripening.

What Should I Have?

Try to choose good fats such as those found in fish, olive oil, flaxseeds, and other nuts and seeds rather than bad fats such as chips and fried foods that add on the weight. Avoid hydrogenated oils and trans fats. Drink healthier beverages like water, teas, and 100 percent fruit juice rather than sodas and sugary soft drinks. Try to avoid high-fructose corn syrup, and even artificial sweeteners.

Choose roasted vegetables and avoid fried vegetables.

ESSENTIAL

Recent studies and research on nutrition and genes suggest that the chemicals in the foods you eat "talk" to your genes. To be sure they are sending out only loud and clear, healthy messages that can help you remain strong, vital, and disease free, health professionals advise people to eat five to ten daily servings of a variety of whole foods every day. Not only fruits and vegetables, but also whole grains, cold-water fish, nuts, and healthy fats like those in olive oil and flaxseed oil.

Try to choose more fish and chicken than red meat. Try to purchase organic meat that is free from antibiotics and hormones. Eat a variety of the leafy greens—don't just stick to the pale iceberg. Experiment with the variety of flavors of the items that can go into a salad. Check the labels on your salad dressings to avoid the additives, or make your own great dressings.

For sweeteners use stevia, honey, pure maple syrup, barley malt, and agave syrup, and avoid corn syrup and white refined sugar.

A Consistent Exercise Plan

Set the time: Most experts agree that the best time to exercise is the morning before work (or before any other family responsibilities). Morning exercise leaves you feeling energized, already proud of your effort and accomplishment, and ready to take on the day. The second best time is immediately after work (before you get home and have other responsibilities or you sit down to rest). Even if you feel tired, do the exercise. Most of the time you will feel better after exercising because you are breathing better, using oxygen, and often there is an exercise "high" that can carry you onward.

Set the places and vary them. If you have a gym between your home and work, stop in; or, the most modest exercise equipment for the home can still give you a good workout. Many exercise professionals agree that giving yourself a variety of exercise plans works for variables in the weather and guards against boredom. Look into an alternating plan that includes weight-lifting, walking, running, tennis, bicycling, aerobics, equipment use, dance classes, Pilates, yoga, swimming, gardening, etc. And housework does count too!

FACT

You can maintain good eating habits even during the holidays, or when on vacation. If you know you are going to have an extra cocktail or two, or a rich dessert, be sure to increase your intake of fruits and greens. Even when vacationing in a land of culinary pleasures, you can always ask for salads instead of potatoes or pasta, and fresh fish instead of meat—and you might be surprised at how wonderfully such things are prepared in different places.

Give yourself motivation if you need it. Some people find great success with making games with their exercise programs. Simple ones are keeping track of distance, times, weight, etc. But there are other games. Some runners figure out how many miles it is to a certain destination, then figure out how far they run in a week and set a target date for reaching their destination. Using a pedometer can work. Pick a number of steps to go—maybe 10,000. Then set your goals to walk so many hundred extra steps a day or week.

Pace Yourself

You don't have to go a long distance all at once, and nobody says exercise has to be ½ hour or an hour at a time. In fact, the more you push yourself over your limit, the more you will be inclined to quit. You can't turn yourself into a marathon-running superstar overnight, but you can certainly build up to it. If you exercise for just ten minutes three times a day, that gives you ½ hour a day. Fitness gurus recommend adding ten-minute bursts of activity during the day, and it all adds up.

Take great note of all your progress and reward yourself for that. Look for things like having better energy, getting better sleep, thinking more clearly, noticing your muscles working easily without pain, and getting a good report from a health professional. Nobody is ever too old to love a reward for putting in effort and work, so decide on what you want—and you'll get it.

ESSENTIAL

The buddy system works for many a thing—and a little socializing while exercising can be both rewarding and motivating. If you have a gym friend or a walking buddy, you're less likely to quit, because you motivate each other to keep going! Besides, who doesn't love a good chat when burning calories?

Remember that exercise helps in these ways:

- Your body gets better at taking in and using oxygen, which helps your cells burn fat better.
- It helps circulation, fueling muscles and the body, and providing better energy.
- It helps weight management by burning calories, keeping your metabolism going strong.
- It improves your physique. Weightlifting can reduce loss of muscle tissue during weight loss, as well as toning and defining.
- Aerobic exercise or cardiovascular keeps your heart rate healthier.

Cleansing Again in the Future

Many people find that as they incorporate healthy foods into their life, their bodies actually speak to them, telling them automatically what to eat and not to eat. Your systems do change, and cravings really can change. There is nothing better than the great feeling you get from feeling strong or rejuvenated, breathing easier, having better digestion, a natural weight, nice skin quality, better concentration, less headaches or pains or stiffness in joints and muscles, better sleep, and better immunity to colds, flues, illnesses, with a more upbeat and positive attitude and a relaxed feeling. You may wish to repeat a cleanse process, trying out a different set of recipes, and setting some new goals.

Future Cleanses

Many cleansers find themselves backsliding, especially around holidays or other notable occasions when food is plenty and they find themselves slipping back into their old bad habits. Doing a cleanse again is a great way to clean house and get back on the track to better health. But it's important to listen to your body, whether it's your first or fiftieth cleanse. You never know how your body will react, so keep a keen ear to what your body needs and what you are giving it.

ALERT

If you did a cleanse before and don't have the fondest memories of it, re-examine why this may be. Did you try to do too much? Were your expectations too high? This time, try another cleanse and set reasonable goals for yourself. You might find the cleanse that's just right for you!

Transition Recipes: Smoothies and Blends for Anytime

These recipes are perfect for transitioning out of your cleanse into your normal diet. Try a few with small meals!

Basic Fruit Mix-and-Match Power Smoothie

This smoothie packs a powerful punch of energy. It gives you the option of choosing tofu, yogurt, or cottage cheese for your protein, so choose whichever texture you prefer.

INGREDIENTS | YIELDS 1–2 SERVINGS

1 cup fresh or frozen fruit of your choice

4 ounces tofu, or 1 cup yogurt, or ½ cup cottage cheese

1 teaspoon ground flaxseed

½–1 banana

2 tablespoons rolled oats, or 2 tablespoons wheat germ

½ avocado

½ cup pomegranate, acai, orange, or apple juice

1 (2-ounce) scoop protein powder

1 cup water, or 1 cup cooled green tea

2–3 ice cubes, as desired for "iciness"

Cinnamon, nutmeg, ginger, to taste (optional)

1–2 tablespoons nuts or seeds (optional)

1–2 dried pitted prunes (optional)

1 cup chopped kale or spinach leaves (optional)

Combine all the ingredients in a blender and blend smooth, pour into a glass and serve.

Easy Waldorf Soup Appetizer

This veggie drink has a delicious taste and nutrients like protein, omega-3s, and iron—all in one glass.

INGREDIENTS | YIELDS 1 SERVING

1 cup chopped spinach leaves

½ tomato, chopped

½ cucumber, chopped

¼ cup pure apple juice, or chopped apple

¼ cup walnuts (chopped or ground will add a bit of crunch, or soak overnight to soften for smooth consistency)

Add all the ingredients to a blender and blend to a nice thickness, pour into a glass and serve.

Chai Protein Smoothie

Who says you have to go to an expensive coffee shop to get a chai? With this recipe you can make a healthier version at home that can keep you going through your post-cleanse day.

INGREDIENTS | YIELDS 1 SERVING

1 cup fat-free milk, or soy milk

1½-inch stick cinnamon

¼-inch piece fresh ginger thinly sliced

6 cloves

6 cardamom pods

⅛ teaspoon ground nutmeg

3 teaspoons tea leaves (or 1 chai tea bag for the quick-preparation method)

Stevia or honey, to taste

1 (2-ounce) scoop protein powder

1. In a saucepan over medium heat, bring the milk and spices to a simmer for 10 minutes.

2. Add the tea leaves; cover, steep for 3 minutes, and then strain. Sweeten to taste and refrigerate.

3. When chilled, blend with protein powder.

4. For the quick tea bag method, bring milk to simmer in a saucepan, or microwave, and then pour over the tea bag and steep.

5. Chill in the refrigerator, then blend with protein powder and add additional spices to taste if desired.

Cold or Hot Tomato Soup Plus Pesto Power

This recipe calls for sage, but if you prefer basil, you can swap the two. It also calls for Parmesan cheese, but if you're not a cheese fan, feel free to swap it for chopped walnuts.

INGREDIENTS | YIELDS 1 SERVING

¼ cup extra-virgin olive oil

¼ cup Parmesan cheese, or 1 cup chopped walnuts

2 tablespoons flaxseeds

2 tablespoons fresh sage or basil

1 clove garlic

1 tablespoon fresh parsley

¼ cup nuts of your choice: pecans, pine nuts, walnuts, almonds

2 cups cilantro leaves

2 tablespoons cider vinegar

1 seeded and chopped jalapeño pepper (optional)

3 tablespoons water

Sea salt, to taste

Blend all the ingredients together in a blender or food processor to smooth, or chunky as desired. Pour into a bowl and serve.

Quick Cold Tomato Soup

*If you prefer your tomato soup hot, you can heat this mixture
after it's been blended for a steamy treat.*

INGREDIENTS | YIELDS 1 SERVING

1–2 tomatoes, chopped

1 stalk celery, strings removed and chopped

2 tablespoons lemon juice

1 sprig fresh basil

1 sprig fresh oregano

1 teaspoon chopped red onion

½ cucumber

½ cup water

Sea salt, to taste

Pepper, to taste

Cayenne, to taste

1 teaspoon honey to sweeten, if desired

Combine all the ingredients and blend in a blender or food processor to smooth or chunky as desired. Pour into a bowl to serve.

Basic Fruit and Veggie Smoothie

For a simple version of this recipe, go minty and refreshing with 1 pear, ½ banana, 1 cup of skim milk that will whip up in a blender to frothy, and add ½ cup fresh mint leaves for that cool green tone.

INGREDIENTS | YIELDS 1–2 SERVINGS

1 pear or peach, pitted or seeded and chopped, or ½ cup green grapes, chopped

½ banana

½ cup pomegranate or blueberry juice

1 cup kale, spinach, collard greens, chopped

1 stalk celery, chopped

½ cucumber

½ avocado

2 sprigs parsley or cilantro

Squeeze of lemon juice

1 cup water

1 teaspoon ground flaxseed

¼-inch peeled and grated gingerroot (optional)

Cinnamon, to taste (optional)

Honey or stevia, to taste (optional)

Place all ingredients in a blender or food processor and blend smooth. Pour into a glass and serve.

APPENDIX

Resource Guide

Resource Guide

Wholly Marcrobiotics

Owned and operated by Gayle Stolove, BS, RN, LMT, Wholly Macrobiotics offers private natural lifestyle counseling/consultations specializing in health-related issues, wholistic diagnosis, seasonal and green consciousness living, macrobiotics, natural foods home delivery services, personal chef services, and more.

www.whollymacrobiotics.com

WebMD

A reliable online source of information on health, fitness, and lifestyle, WebMD offers general health advice, up-to-date and accurate information on various medical conditions, as well as community forums on a long list of health and health-related issues.

www.webmd.com

World's Healthiest Foods

The website of the George Mateljan Foundation for the World's Healthiest Foods. The foundation's founder, George Mateljan, has dedicated his life to discovering, developing, and sharing scientifically proven information about the benefits of healthy eating. The site offers an unbiased, independent perspective of a nonprofit, and also offers practical, simple, and affordable ways to enjoy the healthy foods suggested to fit your individual lifestyle.

www.whfoods.com

Life Extension

Life Extension is a recognized global authority on nutrition, health, and wellness, and is a reliable provider of evidence-based information on antiaging medicine, therapies, and lifestyles.

www.lifeextension.org

The National Center for Biotechnology Information

The website of the National Center for Biotechnology Information, a division of the National Institutes of Health and the National Library of Medicine. It is the authoritative and comprehensive searchable database of published medical research and clinical studies.

www.pubmed.com

The USDA's National Agriculture Library

This site is a service provided by the USDA's National Agriculture Library. It is a gateway to reliable information on nutrition, healthy eating, physical activity, and food safety for consumers as obtained by the federal government.

www.nutrition.gov

The USDA Center for Nutrition Policy and Promotion

The USDA Center for Nutrition Policy and Promotion works to improve the health and well-being of Americans by developing and promoting dietary guidance that links scientific research to the nutrition needs of consumers. The CNPP website is a resource of the USDA's Food, Nutrition, and Consumer Services.

www.cnpp.usda.gov

The American Heart Association's Delicious Decisions

This website offers heart-healthy tips, recipes, and nutritional information from the American Heart Association.

www.deliciousdecisions.org

Dorothy R. Friedman School of Nutrition Science and Policy of Tufts University

This site is a service of the Dorothy R. Friedman School of Nutrition Science and Policy of Tufts University. It provides links to nutrition news and reviews of other nutritional websites.

http://nutrition.tufts.edu/1174562918741/Nutrition-Page-nl2w_1177941613331.html

The Everything® Raw Food Recipe Book, **by Mike Snyder, with Nancy Faass, MSW, MPH, and Lorena Novak Bull, RD (F+W Media, Inc., 2010); visit** *www.adamsmedia.com*

Whether you begin to incorporate raw foods into your diet, or find you love the benefits of raw food, this guidebook gives you 300 amazing recipes from dieticians and nutritionists and a leading expert and keynote speaker on vegan and raw food cuisine and lifestyle. Along with tasty combinations, each easy-to-prepare recipe gives great descriptions of the benefits and particular nutritional punch of the ingredients. The book represents a new wave of thinking in foods.

The Everything® Juicing Book, **by Carole Jacobs and Chef Patrice Johnson, with Nicole Cormier, RD (F+W Media, Inc., 2010); visit** *www.adamsmedia.com*

The purchase of a juicer for your kitchen is a handy gadget that makes drinking delicious, nutritious fruit and vegetable juices a delight anytime. This guidebook provides not only recipes but also descriptions on how particular nutrients in juices can help you ward off colds, aches, and pains, shed pounds, prevent illnesses, and promote anti-aging benefits.

Index

X

Xanthophylls, 99

Y

Yeast, nutritional, 89, 90, 91
Yellow–A Great Color for Squash Soup, 139
Yellow and orange superfoods, 99
Yogurt, 27, 28, 32, 53, 54, 70, 72, 109, 125, 139,
    140, 158, 191, 204, 221, 222, 223, 241

Z

Zinc, 119, 166, 181, 183, 216, 231
Zucchini, 54, 70, 206
    Zuper Soup, 70

We Have
EVERYTHING®
on Anything!

With more than 19 million copies sold, **the Everything® series** has become one of America's favorite resources for solving problems, learning new skills, and organizing lives. Our brand is not only recognizable—it's also welcomed.

The series is a hand-in-hand partner for people who are ready to tackle new subjects—like you!

For more information on the Everything® series, please visit *www.adamsmedia.com*

The Everything® list spans a wide range of subjects, with more than 500 titles covering 25 different categories:

Business	History	Reference
Careers	Home Improvement	Religion
Children's Storybooks	Everything Kids	Self-Help
Computers	Languages	Sports & Fitness
Cooking	Music	Travel
Crafts and Hobbies	New Age	Wedding
Education/Schools	Parenting	Writing
Games and Puzzles	P	
Health	Pets	